ALSO BY THE AUTHOR

POEMS

Something Beautiful Travels Far

Two Women

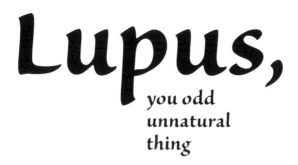

Lupus,
you odd
unnatural
thing

a tale of auto-immunity

Shaista Tayabali

www.lupusinflight.com
Copyright © Shaista Tayabali 2021

Chapter illustrations by Olga, BGBOXXX, Simon Child, Maria Zamchy from the Noun Project

ISBN: 9798777771766
Imprint: Independently published

CONTENTS

for Perveen, who gave me life, my name, and art
&
for Chotu, beloved soulmate, friend of the heart

You don't always have to be doing something.
You can just be, and that's plenty.
—*Alice Walker*

She was already learning that if you ignore the
rules people will, half the time, quietly rewrite
them so that they don't apply to you.
—*Terry Pratchett*

Writing a book is a horrible, exhausting struggle,
like a long bout with some painful illness.
One would never undertake such a thing if one
were not driven on by some demon whom one
can neither resist nor understand.
—*George Orwell*

THE APPOINTMENT
IN SAMARRA

On the last night of 2012, in an arty flat in Singapore, my hostess found me stretching up towards an intriguing title; the shelf in question was too high for me to reach.

Unsurprised by my skulking around, she rescued the tantalising book. She had just read it, she said, and thought I'd like it.

'In fact, here,' she handed it over. 'You have it.'

'Really?' I asked, 'are you sure?'

I was polite and grateful, all the while clutching on to a gift I had no intention of refusing. The book was a paperback, but thick, something to hold on to with both hands. The New Year had yet to be rung in with false merriment and truthful wishes, but I was ready to leave. I have always believed in the purposefulness of books, particularly the ones we don't know we are about to encounter for the first time. The ones that seem to be waiting for us.

The old year was still hanging on by a final thread, when, ensconced in my younger brother Irfan's office-turned-temporary-bedroom for visiting sister, I opened my first book of the new reading year. *The End of Your Life Book Club* by Will Schwalbe is a memoir by a son about the last year of his mother's life, as she walks towards her death from pancreatic cancer. Mother and son hold each other's hands through a series of books they read together in a book club they joined. A book club of two.

I was instantly connected. In the Author's Note, Schwalbe quotes his mother: 'Do your best and that's all you can do.' Words my mother has reiterated throughout our lives. Words that have occasionally driven me to bellow, 'But how can I know what my best is? How will I know? When will I know? Who decides what 'my best' is?'

The first sentence of *The End of Your Life Book Club* begins with coffee: 'We were nuts about the mocha in the waiting room', allaying any fears the reader might have had about a 'cancer book'. A relatable book, you think. And then: 'The coffee isn't so good, and the hot chocolate is worse. But if, as Mom and I discovered, you push the "mocha" button, you see how two not-very-good things can come together to make something quite delicious.' Relatable *and* wise.

By the second paragraph, when we are located 'where people with cancer wait to see their doctors and to be hooked up to a drip for doses of the life prolonging poison that is one of the wonders of the modern medical world', I was hooked.

By the end of 2012, I had been on two different types of IV drips for four years – a selective chemotherapy, or more accurately, a monoclonal antibody therapy, called Rituximab, and Intravenous Immunoglobulins or IVIg, a collection of human antibodies sourced from millions of blood donors; one destroys part of my immune complex pathway and the other invigorates it. Schwalbe's book filled me with happiness. Mothers, literature, illness and dying. The perfect combination.

And then on page 21, Schwalbe quotes *The Appointment in Samarra*, Somerset Maugham's retelling of the classic Iraqi parable in which the servant of a rich merchant, frightened to have come upon Death in a marketplace in Baghdad, borrows the merchant's horse, and flees to Samarra. When the merchant comes upon Death later that same day, he questions her: 'Why did you frighten my servant?' Death explains that the servant had misinterpreted a start of surprise for a threatening gesture. 'I was astonished to see him in Baghdad,' she says, 'for I had an appointment with him tonight in Samarra.'

I read these words, tumbled out of my snuggled sheets, legs fishtailing free, and reached for my iPad. With a sense of urgency, I started typing the first lines of what would become this book. How had I believed there was time enough? There was no more time. The time to begin was now, January 1st, 2013, while the world was still awake and lighting fireworks. Still hopeful.

⁓

It wasn't death I feared was coming for me that night in Singapore or waiting for me as soon as I stepped back into the bitter chill of Heathrow Airport. I had wanted to write this book ever since the first year of my diagnosis. I had known I needed to write it since the day of my diagnosis at eighteen, when I came home from hospital, and immediately searched online for a book that would act as guide and friend. I wanted poetry and truth, wisdom and humour. The book I was looking for did not yet exist. I had thought, at that time, in the way of all teenagers, or perhaps all newly diagnosed patients, that 'it', the mysteriously named illness, would pass, and pass quickly, and then, when the shadow had retreated, I would step into my authorial right to tell my story, and tell it well, with the necessary perspective. With wit, hopefully, and even compassion.

That the years would sandwich together in a hopeless mess of indistinguishable ingredients never occurred to me. I had set myself dates. By twenty-five, I would have written The Book, and published a collection of poetry. By thirty, I would have built a new life for myself, far away from the old, resting like the Cheshire Cat atop my achievements. But when thirty came and death visited again, in passing, like she did the first time, when I was nineteen, I realised I was unafraid of death. Or rather, not inspired enough by the fear of death. There was something else I was more afraid of.

Something that had been breathing the hours with me. Something that had been there with me at my birth, had imprisoned me in bed for three months when I was a child in India, and when I flew thousands of miles away from our first meeting place, it had followed me. Or had it already arrived in England before me? It gave me a few years of seeming freedom, and then never let me go. No matter how far I run, this is always waiting for me. Better to face up to it.

Lupus in fabula. The wolf in the fable. Who speaks of the wolf, conjures the wolf. Who writes of the wolf, may not conquer the wolf, but perhaps she may understand? I write to know the wolf better. I write in an attempt to conquer fear. I write because I believe I am *kintsukuroi*, broken pottery joined by gold dust and lacquer: where the break joins, there is no seamless transition. You can see both the suffering and the mechanism of healing.

I speak of love and the wolf curls its tail. Waiting, watching, between gold dust and shadows, as I begin.

PSSU

Katrina, nurse from Belfast,
remembers me from university.
Dolly, blithe spirit, trills,
'Would you believe I'm 90?'

Louise, with the rare cancer,
talking without a voice box;
Edna, Joan, Quiet Ann,
women, their lives unplanned

for days like these,
days that erase their femininity.

A COLLECTION OF HUMAN MOMENTS IN AN UNEXPECTED PLACE

Until the coronavirus upended global normalcy, I used to receive three weekly infusions of Intravenous Immunoglobulins at the hospital, to bolster my ravaged immune system.

Every few months of the first years of these infusions, Immunology would ask if I wanted to self-inject the immunoglobulins. *Sub cut will make your life so much easier,* they enthused. *Just a couple of hours in your tummy, every week, in the comfort of your own home.*

A nurse gave me a trial stomach injection of 10ml. It hurt, and where the needle invaded, my stomach swelled into a small hillock. *Oh, yes, that happens the first few times, the swellings, the bruises, but then you'll get used to it!*

This was said cheerily, as though she were conferring a gift on me.

The gift of what, exactly? Loneliness?

I like coming into hospital.

There. I said it.

PSSU, which stands for Patient Short Stay Unit, is a little community of friendly faces, wry, deathly humour and sickness gags. I meet people. Occasionally, when I bump into familiar faces, I forget names, but the sense of fellowship once instilled over IVs and beeping motor pumps is impossible to sever. A woman recognized me because the last time we had been in-patients together, I had inflicted a leaf on her with a poem inscribed on it. I had been practicing ninja poetry that day – penning lines from my poems onto autumn leaves and then taping the leaves to the hospital walls. Someone caught me in the act and told me off. Said it wasn't hygienic. I've never done it again. But I might.

My steadfast refusal to switch from IV immunoglobulins to subcutaneous immunoglobulins finally caught the attention of my consultant, who happens to be the Director of the Cambridge Immunology Department. Intrigued, he invited me to share the deeper reason for my insistence. 'I would never have met Clive James, if it weren't for our shared sessions on the ward,' I said, simply. And Clive being his patient too, Dr. Kumar understood. No more discussion on the matter would be necessary, he assured me.

For years, Clive and I met every three weeks, his goblins being infused at a faster pace than mine, but there was always time to compare notes on the matter of books and the matter of death.

Clive made it to his eightieth birthday and died mere weeks before a pandemic virus began disrupting our world. His timing was impeccable. He would have hated being socially distanced from his beloved granddaughter and he would have been forced to be sealed off with his grim assortment of co-morbidities. Planting needles into his own flesh and patiently plunging serum into tissue, as I now do, every week, would have appealed even less. The loneliness I envisaged, years before subcutaneous injections became inevitable for me, was worth postponing. How else would I have trundled my motor pump across the ward to offer the famous Australian critic freshly baked Guinness cake, courtesy of a Marian Keyes recipe? I had baked the cake the night before, a treat for myself, to accompany my copy of her latest novel, *The Brightest Star in the*

Sky. Across cake and Keyes, the kid from Kogarah and I became pals.

Clive's yawns were leonine. He turned the infusion bay into his drawing room by holding no measure of that sound in discretion. Occasionally, in his eagerness to skedaddle home, Clive would forget some portion of his garments. His cardigan. A scarf. But also, his slippers. To stop him shuffling off in his socks, I ahoyed him back. I was as unimpressed by his fashion as he was entertained by mine. His was sixties French philosopher, black, with crumbs. Mine was, is, anything to brighten the spirit. When the carcinomas took a particularly gruesome bite off the top of his head, I offered my olive-green beret. Soft wool and effortlessly stylish, Clive swiped it, without hesitation.

We brought very different books to hospital. Clive was efficient and neat, with one palm sized copy of the essays or poetry of dead, white men. I brought women, writers of colour. I gave him books until I realised that giving books to Clive James was the very definition of taking sand to the Gobi Desert. I did give him my copy of Caitlin Moran's latest collection of essays because he seemed to be eying it covetously but then again, I might have misinterpreted enthusiasm for interest. I gave him passages to read from my copy of *The Good Immigrant*, but I kept the book. We both agreed without ever needing to mention it, that it would be beyond fathoming to come into hospital without at least one book.

I overkill. I arrive with iPad, magazine, and two books. For choice. And if it is a chatty, people filled session, I read very little of any of the delights brought in with me. But leave the house without them, I cannot. I may be listening to an audiobook on my iPad, but I will always have a physical book accompanying me. We also differed on the matter of writing in hospital. Clive didn't. At least he never did so flagrantly, as I do. Writers never cease writing in their heads.

⌒

I don't see as many familiar faces as you might expect after years of regular infusions on the same ward. Maybe we are simply too tired to etch each other onto our mental drawing board. Too much pinned on there.

Some people, of course, are unforgettable. Particularly a certain type of truth telling woman. Working class. Roots gone white at the centre, but otherwise perfectly coiffed. A smoker's cough even though she doesn't smoke. If she were from the American South, she would be at home in a Flannery O'Connor novel.

'That's the trouble with the young ones now,' she opines. 'Don't know how to speak their minds. I say *No More!* now. Since my marriage ended, I've become a different person. When he left me, he wanted to sell the house. So, I took him to court. And I won. The judge told me, it's the smallest little word, *No*, if only people would use it more. You say *No*, Mrs. M, he says, and you'll be just fine.'

She talks about me in a loud voice, meant for my ears and simultaneously, not. She discusses my race and ethnicity. 'Father's English, mother's Indian. Mixed. Been here generations and generations like many of them have.' She adds this so knowledgeably that I am hypnotised – perhaps this is who I am, and I didn't know? She discusses no other patient on the ward, and the ward this Friday is packed. She describes me as lovely, and hardworking, because I am typing furiously. I am tempted to tell her I am writing her down into my book, and since books have the potential to exist for a few forevers, I am writing her down into posterity. But I like to think she knows this already. Hence the carrying voice, and the winking; she winks at me every time she catches my eye. She blends in a non-violent racism with an Everywoman quality that is hard to resist. I don't wink back, since I'm not a person who has ever winked at anyone in her life. (Which eye do you use for the wink? Does it come naturally? Is there a rule?)

The cleaner on the ward is a friendly sort. We have been meeting and greeting one another for all the years I have been coming to this ward. We ask after each other's families. We share snippets of our lives, usually revolving around when we intend to travel or how lovely it was to be with family. We never discuss the weather. I always smile at him. He always smiles at me. I always smile at everyone. They decide if they wish to smile at me.

I was typing, as I said, furiously, so it took a moment to register him standing, waiting, patient sweeper, for me to look up.

I look up. We greet one another in our usual manner. Nod, smile. Nod, smile. He carries on to the next chair. I carry on typing.

From across the room: 'Men are *so* obvious.'
I keep typing. Not looking up.
'Men are so *obvious!*'
I'd been given one more chance. And that was it.
'Did you hear what I said?'

I lift my eyes. My laughing eyes, because she really, really wants my attention. I explain that he is an old friend. A decent man, good husband and father. We have been greeting each other for many years.

'I take your point,' she says, not taking anything. 'But did you see the way he just hung around you, waiting for the pretty girl to look up?'

Women try to tell each other things but we seem unable to speak and listen at the same time. We seem incapable of learning in sync. There is very little space for a thirty-year old to truly hear the lessons and experiences of a seventy-year old. Media does not provide the space, and, in the personal equation, the conversation is deafened by the endless negotiation of figuring out how to reconfigure the kind of woman you want to be. There is so much to unlearn that we can never quite catch up with what needs to be newly learned.

She knows she is going to die. Only a quarter of a lung left. 'I want to die in my bed. Just go to sleep and never wake. No better way to go, is there?'

Her feet are swollen but she hasn't the energy to press the button that will lift her footrest up. She hasn't the energy to lean back in her chair. She is poised, arms tucked into her sides, a scrawny, soothsaying elf.

I go to the bathroom, trailing my IV with me. As I'm finishing up, I overhear someone making noisy, humorous goodbyes. By the time I return to the ward, she is gone. This is the way of it. She never told me her name. I was never asked mine. We might recognise each other if we were to meet again on opposite sides of this ward. But would we know each other in the outside world?

When I try to write fiction, this is my dilemma: I know my characters in the middle of their lives. Suddenly I come upon them. I can hear them speak, see them struggle. I can set a scene. Dialogue is sparky. But beginnings and endings escape me. Who are they? Where did they come from and where are they going? It's a mystery and attempting to unravel that mystery is the reason I chose to do my MA in Creative Writing, instead of burying myself further in literary academia. I wanted to learn the craft of taking the listening and giving it a structured home. I deliberately set out to do a Masters in writing fiction, and ended up writing a book about my life, because my life is peopled with characters I want to portray just as they are, or at least, as they seem to me.

⌒

When I read Albert Espinosa's *The Yellow World*, I experienced a strange jealousy that cancer patients seem to have their own world in fiction and reality (fellow 'Eggheads' – Espinosa's term), a byword for a certain kind of hell-in-life, a snug, shared snark. But I think I do have that, to a less intense extent, here on PSSU.

I met a young man who could easily have been Albert Espinosa in disguise. He was freshly graduated and didn't mind letting everyone know he was now part of The First Class Honours brigade. *Me too!* I wanted to boast, but it was his moment. He was very cool in a Cool

Patienty sort of way, showing off the expensive diabetes contraption attached to his flesh. We discussed the possibility of subcutaneous infusions, and, being an expert, he had some good advice about it. He talked a mile a dozen, but what I really envied was his life in his usual hospital, on his usual ward. *Everyone knows each other. We've all been coming there for years. We have the same three nurses. It's brilliant!* And then he drops the real gem – they're allowed to manage their own drips. We aren't allowed to manage our medication on the infusion bay. How green I felt. How green with envy.

Sometimes the banter is between nurse and patient. And sometimes the wit is slightly precarious.

'You shouldn't write in books,' says my nurse. 'It ruins it for others.'

'I'm on the fence about it,' I say.

'There's no point. It spoils it for others.'

'But it's my book.'

'But it won't be for long. In the end you're going to...' We look at each other. She follows through, because not to do so would be against her persona, the one she has cultivated in here – '...die. You can't take it with you.'

'Ah, but I'll leave it behind, and those who love me will see their beloved Shaista's writing and feel happy, the way I do when I see my aunt's writing.' (In her copy of *Jane Eyre*, I think, but don't say.)

'You've put on half a kilo,' she says, next. 'Christmas weight gain!'

Death and weight. We've covered the important topics. After this, she becomes kinder. It's the pattern she has patented. And because I have experienced the kindness behind the joking insensitivities, I engage in the duel.

Some days, though, I am so tired I can't be my best hospital self.

Like that's a thing.

But it is a thing because I've made it a thing. I see it reflected around me. We try to be cheerful and humorous to keep the staff going, to keep up each other's morale. We smile knowingly at each other. Implicit is the acceptance that we are here for one another, but we can't talk, not yet. The clear or murky fluids drip into our veins. Some of us sleep. Some have gadgets. Occasionally, a paperback makes a surprising cameo.

The stories write themselves on PSSU.

I take pictures in my head of nurse-patient interactions. There's an art project here, a best-selling book, waiting to happen: *A Collection of Human Moments in An Unexpected Place.*

An old man had a nice, gentle energy about him the other day. Nodding at me, smiling patiently. I'm here, his smile offered. I couldn't take his gift of temporary friendship for several hours. I curled into my blanket, buried my face in my pillow. Amanda Palmer through my earphones. My heart cantankerous at 84bpm, then 96. My head swarmy, swampy. Bees in my head. Trying to listen to my own thoughts. Forced to listen to the bee-beep beeping around me.

Finally, I turn to him. With each question and answer, we piece ourselves together for each other. We get each other. We are each other.

He is seventy-one. He has Wegener's granulomatosis. He is on Rituximab, like me; it's working the best of all the drugs for him, like it is for me. We've been through the same hoops.

'Isn't it impossible to answer the question, *How are you?*' I ask him.

'Impossible,' he agrees. 'How long have they got? They'll never ask us again.'

How are you? We're fine! We say this in unison, chortling together. Like we're in a pub or having a pot of tea in a warm kitchen, biscuit tin at the ready.

'Do you bruise?' I ask.

'All the time,' he says.

'And then,' he continues, 'they say – *But you don't look sick!*'

I am about to tell him about the website dedicated to that phrase, but I refrain. 'I have glaucoma,' I say, instead.

'Me too,' he says.

Turns out we share the same doctor. We extol Keith's virtues for a while.

He pulls up his rucksack off the floor and rummages around. He produces his prescriptions, thicker than mine. I read them, a witness. I am familiar with many of the treatments. He shows me little pots of pills for morning, afternoon, night.

They've taken bone from his hip to replace eaten away bone from his ear. He talks, I listen. I hear the lilt of Cork in his accent. He tells me his name. Michael. 'A good, solid name,' I say. He agrees. He is round faced and ruddy cheeked, which almost lends him a healthy glow. Almost. If I didn't know better, I might say, 'But you don't look sick!' But I know better. He's on steroids. It turns all of us into ruddy-faced hamsters.

There's more. He loves India. He worked near Bombay for a company that my grandfather Rustom worked for. His mother's people are from Cahir, Tipperary, where a friend of mine lives. Where I have been. His father was from Limerick. He has people in Boston, in the Bronx. His niece has lupus, too. (He has heard of lupus!)

Our immigrant and patient tales converge and diverge so naturally it's as though we don't need to meet again. What will there be to say? Haven't we said all that matters already?

Like most patients on Rituximab, he is somehow able to tolerate the fastest rate of infusion. 400 mg/h. 'Doesn't your heart explode at that speed?' I ask.

'I didn't feel so good the last time,' he confides.

His transport arrives.

He gathers his bits and pieces together, looks around in case he has missed anything. He leans down to me. I place my hand in his and we wrap our spare hands around our clasped ones. 'Goodbye, my girl,' he says. Or was it, 'God bless, my girl?'

I forget now, as I wait for someone who loves me, to come be my transport, and carry me home.

⌒

The dots connect over and over again when you live long enough to see the circles, the looping friendliness of human connections. As much as I forget, I remember. Sometimes my mother will remind me of an incident from the wards. *Remember when you gave your slippers away to that woman?* I can't remember. *Remember when you left money under the pillow for the Ponds cream lady?* Yes, her I remember, because I wrote her into a poem.

Dolly had been on the same ward for months. She had been an in-patient in one hospital, then another for years. The hospital staff didn't know what to do with her. She had no one to call her own, and no one seemed to be prepared to take the responsibility of sending her back home. A gentle dementia had settled in. Her world had shrunk to the parameters of a single bed behind a blue paper curtain. She was proud of her skin: *Would you believe I'm 90?* her merry refrain. She had always been a Ponds girl, like her mother. She had no money of her own. I couldn't bear the thought that she could buy nothing from the trolleys that trundled past her twice a day. A small injustice I could remedy before I was discharged. I tucked money under her pillow.

I don't know what became of Dolly. I never know what becomes of my fellow in-patients. I have to leave them in the hands of the unknown, and trust.

One night, when my inability to tolerate the rate of Rituximab fast enough had resulted in an overnight stay, I met Terry. She had a shell-shocked look about her that I recognized instantly. Nothing can prepare you for being dehumanised if you are used to a certain way of life. Being a woman in control. Running the household, feeding the children, minding the husband.

We talk.

She is a dinner lady; her husband works with CCTV. One day, she sees a line appear across her right eye. Things go dark below that line. A little later, the same darkness above the line. Now she is blind. She visits the GP who sends her to an ophthalmologist. She is told it is either multiple sclerosis or optic neuritis. Of the two diagnoses, she is told MS is the better option. She has an MRI scan. All clear. The eye surgeon feels sure this is a one-off and tells her in July that this will not happen again. She need only be vigilant. But of what, he is unable to say. Visual disturbances, she supposes. I meet her in December. The first thing I notice, when she changes into a matching set of pyjamas with a sleeveless top, is how fit she looks. How toned her arms. She looks ready for a run.

She is ready to run. She has been administered intravenous steroid infusions as well as swallowing 60mg of oral prednisone daily. She wants to break out of her skin like a Marvel superhero. She is growing teeth and claws she never knew she possessed. She can feel them growing. *I'm becoming so horrible*, she confides. She tells me, guiltily, of the loveliness of the four men in her life: she has three, sweet sons. She wonders how I am able to be cheerful, buoyant even. She tells me I look younger than my years.

I am meeting myself every time I encounter a stranger on the ward with that shell-shocked, vacant expression. It's like they've pressed the pause button and are waiting for someone to press rewind.

I am living proof that the rewind button does not exist.

And every time the forward button is pressed, things get cumulatively worse. Or as Lily Tomlin said, 'Things have to get a whole lot worse before they get worse.'

They don't know that. Yet.

I seem to represent a peculiar but particular kind of comfort. The comfort of coping. If they knew how long it took me to learn, would all comfort dissipate?

THE NOVICE

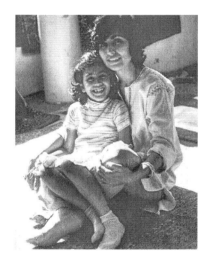

The Fire Within

Let me see if I can make poetry of this.
Let me see if I can whisk fear out of this

'Scintillating Scotoma' – I like the way it fits
the visual fire, the zig zagging
iridescent, shimmering quagmire of this.

Hold still, my whirling dervishes,
so I can count you, claim you, calm you.
Hold still, so I can draw you, close.

We aren't the first to do this.

TELL ME YOUR STORY

When I tell people I am a writer, a poet, they exclaim and appear to be impressed or pleased to have met such a curiosity on an ordinary day.

But then, almost immediately on the heels of their pleasure and surprise, comes this question: 'Are you published?' Taxi drivers, delivery-men, random persons-on-buses, people who openly declare their utter lack of interest in the act of reading want to know if I'm published. I imagine if my answer was, 'Yes! I can be found on a bookshelf in your local bookstore' or 'Yes! In fact, I am carrying a few copies of my book right here, with me, in my handbag. Cash will be fine' might elicit the same response as a gritty, 'Afraid not yet, but I'm hoping to be': a swift change of topic.

When I tell people I have lupus, there is a similar Pavlovian set of responses.
1) Blank look.
2) 'What's that? I've never heard of it.' (As though their ignorance proves lupus cannot possibly exist. Or perhaps it exists only because I just made it up.)
3) 'Lupus... I think I've heard of it. What's it about? What happens to you?'

4) 'Oh, I'm sorry to hear that. I know someone who has it.'

4 can be subdivided into

    a) 'I know someone who has it but they're doing really well now. Have you tried...?' (Insert here all manner of alternative therapies, diet suggestions, exercises.)

    b) 'I know someone who has it. She's always struggling, poor thing.'

    5) 'Well, at least you don't have cancer/AIDS/ALS' (or whichever disease this person finds particularly terrifying.)

    6) Swift change of topic.

And once, in a car, so I couldn't run away:

    7) 'What's your prognosis? Can you die from it? Do you know how long you've got?'

If my fellow in conversation is also a fellow sufferer, they will ask a question of genuine interest, such as, 'How long have you had it? When/how did it start?' In other words, my origin story. Lupus gives us two lives. The one we had before we fell ill/were diagnosed and the one forever after.

Unless, of course, lupus was there with you at your birth. And maybe even before. My mother developed a rash when she was pregnant with me, her face flushed into a red balloon, and her gynaecologist suggested she start eating boiled, bland food because the rashes were unpredictable. My mother remembers this pregnancy as the troublesome one, the one about denial and discomfort, but photographs of her during this pregnancy reveal her joy. Those were the days before ultrasound scans and yet she says she knew I'd be a girl, because she longed for a daughter. Although I cast spells of mysterious rashes and swellings, I grew and survived and began to be a person who needed a name, so I could begin my story.

Don't think of it as a memoir, my older brother Rizwan advises me as I begin the writing of this book. Memoir is a trap. Think of it as a book. I agree, but I cannot escape memoir.

Memoir is the retelling of personal history drawn from memory. A chronic illness patient must provide a memorised narrative of their history every single time they encounter a new doctor in or out of the emergency room. 'Tell me your story, in your own words,' the doctor will encourage you. If your diagnosis was made a year ago, or if you don't have a multi-system, auto-immune disease with fourteen co-morbidities, perhaps you stand a chance of providing this narrative without wanting to gnaw your knuckles off first.

But if you were a child when the first symptoms began, and with them the cycle of injections and hospitalisations, and then a teenager when you were diagnosed, and if your story began in India and wound its way to England, your narrative will be long, complicated, repetitive and unwieldy. The thought of regurgitating this for the twentieth year in the ER while I am wracked with the chills that accompany fever, is enough to make me want to drop to the floor and roll under the emergency room stretcher, face palming all the while.

But I am usually already attached to an IV drip trying to plump up my veins with saline, making it impossible to pull ninja moves without the tedium of blood spurting out of my aggrieved, cannulated arm. So, I take a deep breath, try to avoid cracking a joke ('how long have you got, ha ha?') and get busy with story time. 'Once upon a time when my mother was pregnant with me...' or 'It all began with mouth ulcers, around the age of nine...' or 'I was diagnosed at eighteen, but I was first hospitalised at ten...'

I never tell it the exact same way. I try to keep things interesting, for myself, at least. As a writer, I am perennially afraid of striking boredom into my audience. Words are my métier. I know I am being judged on my performance but there is something else being judged, something that lies beyond my ability to create interest, intrigue, suspense. There are interruptions, for a start. Always off-putting for the dramatist. Mid rehashed memoir, the doctor reaches for my pulse, or a nurse comes into the room with apologies, or a beeper beats me to a punchline of particular significance. My performance is only part theory. There is a practical to follow.

The whole encounter is called an examination and must be treated with the seriousness reserved for examinations. A patient must always be on guard, prepared to answer questions, when often all we want to do is curl into ourselves, shut down unnecessary avenues of energy expenditure and be quiet enough to heal. But we are not in a place conducive to self-healing. We are here to be healed. External healing begins with what we tell doctors, who expect us to follow this principle: what you reveal, we can heal.

Hospitals require us to talk on command. Be examined, questioned and then re-questioned. And then again, and again. Until you know you have tripped yourself up and your memories are lapping over each other and accuracy fled somewhere between the first nurse who took a brief history and this latest medical student who is prepared to give you more time than you knew a doctor was capable of sharing. They are genuinely curious, asking the sort of questions you will later dream your consultant would ask, and you sit in a stupor, because you had only just brought your narrative down to a nifty bullet pointed exercise in brevity. And you did this through trial and error of improvisational theatricality, because unlike medical students who learn how to take a case history, and how to deliver a case history, we, patients, are fumbling around in the murky murk of our own re-tellings.

I never know which snippet from my oral memoir will interest my audience. Sometimes it is the revelation that I am a poet. Even 'writer' may spark an awakening in the indifferent eyes gathering me in.

Sometimes the mention of 'India', or more specifically 'Bombay' – 'oh, you don't call it Mumbai?' – other times, nothing. No hint of applause. Deflated, the poet-storyteller wishes she could wave away her ungrateful listeners and contemplate a fresh approach. But now comes insult to injury. Lift up your top, pull down your jeans, open your eyes wide, stick out your tongue. Say 'aah'. After all those linguistic gymnastics, say 'aah'. How old am I again? In hospital, before a doctor, you are not in control of anything, not even your age.

'Tell me your story, in your own words,' the doctor invites. Tell you who I am? Who am I? I end up looking into the doctor's face for the answer to that question. Why wouldn't I? Doctors hold mysterious powers, we are told; we are sent to their headquarters and instructed to wait for them. They hold the cards with the questions and hold, or withhold, the answers. The computer faces the doctor. Occasionally, when in a charitable mood, a doctor might turn the screen at a slight angle to share something with me – but even with their best intention, I do not possess the sharp eyesight necessary to read either at the distance or the speed before the screen is whisked away from any visible angle. *What does it say???!?* I want to shriek, in full on banshee mode, hair wrapped around fists, but I maintain the norms. Imagine the speed at which I'd be committed to psychiatry if I gave in to that impulse. As it is, my face is constantly being read by others. For what? I cannot tell.

Doctors are the power brokers of my life.

I exist in a state of tension that permeates my life while I wait, in waiting rooms and at home, between appointments. I don't hit peak high blood pressure levels like some people do, but just as I took my school life seriously, so I respond as obediently to code words like 'examination' and 'examination room'.

'Do you mind if I...?' the doctor asks. The patient's acquiescence is a mere formality. The patient knows that any hedging is useless, maybe even dangerous, because you will be considered to be obstructing procedure. Non-compliant. Emotional. 'Patient would not permit...'

There is something chilling about hospital notes – there is always a discrepancy between the emotional, or physical reality of the patient and the recorded case of the doctor or nurse in charge. 'In charge' being the operative phrase because the patient is patently not in charge. To be a patient is to be the object of an action. The moment you are 'admitted' – an interesting word in itself, suggesting your truth has been confirmed by an authority that decides (admits) there is something wrong with you – you are simultaneously legitimised and treated as hospital property, evidenced by the plastic band snapped around your wrist. You have a hospital number and that is your identity – your relevant identity.

There are boxes to be filled or ticked. Spaces left blank. And everything in black and white, filed away for posterity. You are on record. Your truth ceases to matter. The notes hold their own truths – written words appearing as recorded law.

There can be uses to this. Susanna Kaysen, author of the bestselling memoir *Girl, Interrupted* acquired her hospital notes by employing a lawyer. The notes validate her story. But they also condemn her. Kaysen appears to acquiesce to her incarceration by doing nothing to prevent it.

When I think of my own descent down the rabbit hole, I know I did nothing to prevent any of it. Like Kaysen, I was a teenager, and I wasn't given a choice. I wasn't asked if I minded being pumped full of IV grams of Methylprednisone. *They* inserted a cannula and administered the drugs. *They* may say they were saving my life. They may be right. But those initial doses of steroids upset the fine balance of intra-ocular pressure in my eyes and I developed glaucoma. To this day, my diagnosis of steroid-induced glaucoma often has a question mark beside it because no one wants to, or needs to, take responsibility for definitively connecting one action to its devastating consequence. I have lupus. I have glaucoma. So what? There might be another culprit. The very first drug I was prescribed – Hydroxychloroquine or Plaquenil – is now known to cause eye disease.

Who gets to tell this story? Whose story is this? My data exists for anyone to read within the hospital context, and they write me as they see me, not as I wish to be seen. Most of the time I never know which version of the story is being told. The real question here is one of veracity and accuracy – how do you make something true? How do you tell it true? How can you know if it is true? I am rewriting history because my story is fundamentally different depending on who is telling it.

Meanwhile, our appetite for lawyers and doctors on a TV show or in a movie seems endless.

How doctors think, and how doctors feel, is a source of constant fascination played out in documentaries, reality TV, bestselling books. The theatricality of the courtroom is mirrored in the emergency room. Surgeries are called theatres because once upon a time they offered spectacles. Perhaps they still do. Despite the performative streak required of me when relating my medical history, I rarely recognise myself in hospital TV shows. Or movies featuring a hospital episode as the dramatic interlude. Drama is not my experience. Waiting rooms are my experience. Hours of loneliness to fill, in a ward, on a bed.

The irony is that patients make for excellent drama on a TV show, but only as accents in the lives of the heroic beings in white coats and blue or green scrubs. There is a reason that a panoply of shows called 'Patients' or 'Waiting Rooms' doesn't exist. We are the muesli of the hospital. Necessary fodder, but not exactly appetizing. Even when a stroke of the dramatic curses us, it is only the beginning of a long fall down the rabbit hole.

We are not the heroes. We are not the ones conducting the diagnostics or the investigations. Even when a doctor is an anti-hero, he is still the hero.

The first time some people encountered lupus was through a long running gag on the American TV show 'House'. Hugh Laurie can be forgiven most things, but I am not sure this is one of them. The hilarity rested on the possibility of lupus being a catch all for any truly complex, indecipherable combination of symptoms, and then the joke: 'It's not lupus.'

Cancer has reached a unique status in our society; known to most of us, it is almost familial. In 2012, when comedian Tig Notaro made cancer the focus of her stand-up comedy at the Largo Club in Los Angeles, it shocked her audience, because cancer is still The Big C, but her honesty was also met with warmth and applause. An audio recording of that show resulted in a Grammy nomination. Lupus does not have such standing in our community. The joke falls flat for the lupus patient because no one fears the disease enough to need humour as a salve. If your friend's introduction to lupus is the brilliance of Hugh Laurie's wit, tap dancing on the thing that threatens your life, you find yourself in the unenviable position of having to explain that the joke is not a joke. You will do this humourlessly, your mouth set in a grim line, determined not to let the magical memory of Bertie Wooster seduce you into getting the joke after all.

The first thing you ever read about lupus post diagnosis is not an excerpt of a 'House' episode. It is this: *Lupus is incurable.*

The idea is to shock us into awareness and create a public profile prepared to raise funding so a cure can be found. For the newly diagnosed, this is a blow from which a part of us never recovers. It is also a profoundly confusing discovery to make, because the first thing you hear at the moment of your diagnosis is often this: *You have a mild case of lupus. So mild, you probably won't even notice it.*

There are things doctors said to me in the first years of my illness that still impact me today. Repetition is a flaw in writing, but lupus is a repetitive disease. It is a constant literary and medical challenge to free myself from the trap of repetition. If this were a novel, I would include a sequence in which my protagonist made a poignant speech about the fact that twenty years had passed with her walking into the same room in the Rheumatology department of the same hospital in which she was diagnosed. My character would be given the uninterrupted space and the perfect words to describe that reality. It would move the listening consultant to tears (I would write in those tears) and hopefully illuminate something to my reader.

I could write such a speech now. But even if I memorised the words, it would never happen in life, the way I could make it happen in fiction.

The fact that I can empower my character-self in a novel, but can't do it for myself in real life, breaks something in me and makes me equally determined to fix the broken pieces. I want to create those illuminations outside of a novel. I don't know if my experiment will work. I just want to try.

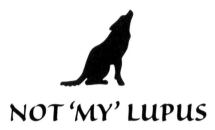

NOT 'MY' LUPUS

The word 'patient' derives from the root 'to suffer'. Patience is thought to be an inherent quality of goodness, attributed most often to saints. The rarity of saints among us is telling.

It can also be an admonition: 'Have patience!' or 'Be patient!'

Lack of the quality can be a judgment on our morality. Particularly if we are women. But equally, so can an abundance of it. 'You are too patient!' As though to suggest a bit of impatience might be a good thing, an indication of passion rather than acquiescence. Authority over submission.

Apart from the saints, who need to suffer in order to translate that suffering into joy, nobody wants to be a patient. Doctors generally want to become doctors. And even when pressured by family, there are no guarantees that you will become a doctor. It is a noble profession to aspire to, and once accomplished, you become the symbol of aspiration for others, belonging in a continuum spanning millennia.

Not so much for the other side on the healing see-saw. Illness is an ignoble state of being for the most part, so we are encouraged to deny, destroy or overcome dis-ease. The acute patient may walk away with no lasting judgment. The chronic illness patient always suspects a personality is being built up around them.

To escape the various stigmas, we are supposed to vociferously state that we are not our illnesses – an illness is a diagnosis and we are so much more than that. It goes against the social narrative to identify or define yourself with illness. But what if I do? I don't mind having 'the' lupus. I mean, of course I mind having lupus, I just don't mind the use of the definite article. What I have a scrappy attitude towards is the nosy interference of the possessive 'my'. It is not 'my' lupus. It's just lupus. Glaucoma. Vasculitis. Pleurisy. Hypothyroidism. I neither invented these diagnoses nor am I reinventing them. I belong to a statistic of millions. And knowing my own history of illness, I also know how easy it is to hold other titles. My first flare of lupus as a child in India was diagnosed as a case of rheumatic fever because of the presentation of high fever, joint pain and tachycardia. It was a tentative diagnosis, much like my first diagnosis in England of suspected enteric fever. And even after sophisticated immunological screening confirmed lupus, over the years various doctors have questioned this. Subacute bacterial endocarditis, malaria and tuberculosis still hover in the expectant air around the Infectious Diseases team.

And yet we are encouraged to personalise disease, to think of it as ours, the medical rationale being that no two auto-immune cases are identical since the genesis for these conditions lie in our DNA. It is also an attempt to enable patient empowerment, to encourage the 'expert patient', an oxymoron for myriad reasons, not least because who volunteers to be an expert at being sick? The expertise of being a patient is a condition thrust upon us.

Who am I as an individual lupus patient? What does it mean to be a unique case worthy of attaching a possessive 'my'? There is no protocol set in place for an individualised treatment plan beyond shifts in dosage. Every lupus patient is told the disease affects each of us uniquely, but we are also told we must follow the only available treatments, none of which are uniquely designed for multi-system immunodeficiency. We are informed that this or that drug causes little to no side effects in other patients. Who are these saints? you wonder, already alienated. A brief foray into any forum and a different truth is revealed by your fellow sufferers. One that makes you quake in anticipation. Patient solidarity is a concept I readily embrace. Patient empowerment is less of a reality.

I cannot divide or subtract myself from the biological misunder-standing that exists in a few of my genes. The intellectual confusion that creates the chaos that is auto-immunity is embedded in every cell of my body. And since mind and brain are part of that equation, perhaps some measure of my thought process is also mis-educated in certain ways. I have little fear in acknowledging the presence of lupus everywhere that is recognisably and also invisibly me. I am attached to this reality without terror. But also, without possessiveness. I do not desire lupus. I did not invite it to stay. But it has staying power. And its address of residence is my body. I am its host. It hosts itself in me, an undesirable immunological reality.

While I do not accept the idea that I must, with every breath, fight this abnormality, something is being fought every day. Or most days. Something that provokes the encouragement of others to adjure me to, 'Fight, Shaista! Fight!'

But people don't realise they are also saying, 'Fight Shaista'. Because the fight is taking place inside Shaista whether she is thinking fighting thoughts or not. Lupus is auto-immune. Instead of producing antibodies that attack pathogens (bacteria, viruses), a system that protects most human beings on an almost continual basis, my body makes auto-an-tibodies. Self-attacking soldiers. The most vital line of defence turns inwards and my body attacks itself.

I dislike the use of metaphor in illness. How can I describe lupus as a civil war in my body when actual civil wars have far more wide-reach-ing catastrophic consequences? The auto-immune battalions of lupus are microscopically contained in my five-foot, two-inch body. A vessel I can carry up the stairs to a comfortable bed. Close my door, tunnel into a duvet, play music. And give thanks for safety. Freedom. Warmth. Eyes shut, my mind is free to open doors I choose. Roam aimlessly or specifically. And return, when I choose.

And yet. The civil war metaphor has at least some basis of parallel logic.

There is another metaphor faced by the lupus patient: an unavoidable one, since it is contained in the name of the diagnosis itself. We are so desperate for clues that we will describe 'our' disease as the wolf within us, hoping some ancient secret will reveal itself. Doctors do not speak to us in this language of metaphor. Their ancestors placed the linguistic burden of wolves upon us, but it is we alone who bear it. The Infectious Diseases consultant who first diagnosed me at eighteen, failed to mention the etymological history I had now inherited, and so did the Rheumatology consultant he transferred me to. The history, nonetheless, seeks us out.

According to Professor Laurent Arnaud from the National Reference Centre for Autoimmune Diseases of Strasbourg, France, the metaphorical wolf first arrives in the year 850 AD with a man named Eraclius, the twenty-fifth Bishop of Liège, who was very ill with 'la loup', so called 'because it eats the flesh'. The first mentions of lupus in the early twelfth and late thirteenth centuries referred to a malignant ulceration destroying the nose or face, and particularly the lower limbs.

Why lupus? The disease mirrored the rapacity of a wolf attack. The Oxford English Dictionary references lupus in a text dated c.1590: 'very hungry like unto a woolfe', most likely quoting the Swiss physician, Paracelsus. In 1776, Daniel Turner, author of 'De Morbis Cutaneis' wrote this: 'if it seize upon the Legs and Thighs, it is termed *Lupus*, the Wolf; for that it is, say some, of a ravenous Nature, and like that fierce creature, not satisfy'd but with Flesh'. Turner defined lupus as 'a cancer of the lower limbs'.

In the 1840s, the Viennese physician, Ferdinand von Hebra, made notes on a distinctive rash 'mainly on the face, on the cheeks and nose in a distribution not dissimilar to a butterfly'. From wolf to butterfly in a few hundred years.

Today, the term 'lupus vorax' or 'vulgaris' is obsolete; the malignant ulceration referred to what doctors now recognize as cutaneous tuberculosis. Medical confusion, however, continued for centuries, and records of female patients are almost entirely absent from these medieval archives.

In 1851, Pierre Cazenave, a Parisian dermatologist, combined lupus, the Latin word already in existence, with a Greek-rooted French word, érythémateux, from erythrocytes or red blood cells. Later, érythémateux was Latinized to erythematosus and, since the condition affected various other parts of the body – heart, lungs, kidneys, joints, nervous system – 'systemic' prefixed 'lupus erythematosus'. Systemic Lupus Erythematosus is weighty but informative. The reduction to 'lupus' is not helpful in explaining the disease, so we return to metaphor. To animals. To shadows. Even to the stars.

Lupus and cancer share a Latinate origin, bound by astronomy; they are constellations possessing a startling beauty at a certain time of night. But here is the difference: the lupus patient forms an instant connection with wolves. The Wolf becomes the metaphor that holds our psyche and our afflicted flesh together. Do cancer patients anthropomorphise crabs? Only once have I come across the crab used as external metaphor – in Paul Kalanithi's exquisite memoir *When Breath Becomes Air*. Kalanithi writes: 'As desperately as I now wanted to feel triumphant, instead I felt the claws of the crab holding me back.'

I've read countless cancer memoirs. They are the closest reference point for the world I live in, even though the most significant difference – the difference that makes all the difference – is that everyone has heard of cancer, fears or respects cancer, and no one fears or respects lupus. It is not an awe-inspiring disease. Cancer is The Big C. Lupus cannot decide if it is The Big L or the little l; it feels like the poor relative of a richer disease – the one who has to suffer silently because there is nothing interesting about being poor.

There is a casual association of criminality in the possessive 'your' cancer or 'your' lupus. A light suggestion that it is 'your' fault. 'Your' problem. Part of the decoding undertaken by the detective doctor is trying to ascertain what exactly is the fault of lupus, or what may be ascribed to lifestyle, personality, factors of stress and environment. I am regularly asked by doctors if I think it is lupus at work or something else. When I am made assistant detective, language fractures even further since I believe there is no separation between lupus and 'something else'. My body houses a particular set of genes, which code themselves into complex immune pathways that are eventually felt or seen as symptoms.

I fantasise about a department I have invented in my mind. The Department of Auto-Immunity. In this department I am whole, and there is a hive of minds at work on the relationship between genetics, immunology and the uniquely coded sequence that causes self to attack self. But the medical world is not queuing up to discover a cure for lupus. Lupus is not a byword for research or funding.

⌒⌐

And so, even with the conscious awareness that I am not a wolf, that I know almost nothing about wolves, ask me how it feels.

How does it feel?
Like there's an animal inside of me. Or I am animal. These are the werewolf moments:

I'll be sitting in the car with my sweet parents in the front, my mother describing the quaintly dressed woman on the other side of the road for my father's amusement, or both of them discussing the recent antics of their grandchildren, and I, at the back, strapped in for safety, am thirsting for blood, red eyed and frantic. A contained fury, I grit and grip my teeth, curl my claws into my palms and breathe into the hell.

They are no fools, these sweet parents of mine. They have lived with this wolf-child-woman for as long as I have, and they know exactly what to do.

Nothing.

They neither invite the wolf to speak nor deny him the right to spit and hiss. Him? Her? It is a genderless beast.

Revved up, and nowhere to go, I am a morass of invisible drum-beats. Throbbing pulse, da-dum-dum-dum. Swelling lymph nodes, ba-bum-bum. Roiling nausea, tarum-pum-pum. Left eye migraine, kerrash-kerrack. Fever, fever, fever.

I don't burst. I don't explode and shatter into broken Shaista cells that can be gathered up by my parents, and tenderly re-moulded with love, sunshine and flowers into a new, glowing self. There is no imme-diate restoration to be had. But the years have taught me to cling to one thing – the voice in my head that is translating the experience into language. The words themselves are not the solution, but the act of writing in my head, the knowledge that my future self's fingers will scribe with pen, will type into the whiteness, the blankness, the beautiful blackness of letters. A poem. A line. My own. Or perhaps belonging to some other animal-soul in terror.

We borrow language from each other. We remember stories, punch-lines, moralities and also that there are no punchlines, moralities, end-ings. It goes on. This is how I go on. The words. Writing. The sharp tearing and through the slit, a memory of something pure, neither human nor animal, but natural. An instinct. Survival.

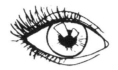

THE HABIT OF SEEING

I have a vivid imagination.

Sometimes it is the trick of my mind. More often, it is the trick of my eyes.

Does this ever happen to you: you're looking at a sheet, slightly crumpled on the bed, and instead of fabric creases, you see a face? A recognisable face? Strong, clean features. Aquiline nose. Hooded sockets. No eyes. The no-eyes give it away, force me to un-focus and bring me back to the sheet.

In the fold of a curtain, do you see the profile of a bearded man? I sketch him onto paper. As I trace the last of his curls, I look up, blink and he is gone, leaving only a pattern of roses.

Or I see a beautiful sculpture. A Henry Moore, or a Barbara Hepworth. When I ask my friend what she thinks of the art, she says it isn't a Moore. It's an old water pump. Go take a closer look, she suggests. I walk the eighteen feet to the object and discover the pump. And I become two people. The person who saw an unexpectedly uplifting stone sculpture in an old English pub, and the one looking at an equally historical piece of manmade work. Both objects are beautiful, but the beauty resides not so much in the object as in the fact that I see, twice.

In textbook speak, I have Charles Bonnet syndrome, but it is this haiku by Wendy Cope that truly encapsulates much of my visual experience:

What's that amazing
new lemon-yellow flower?
Oh yes, a football.

The title of the haiku reveals its meaning: 'Looking Out of the Back Bedroom Window Without My Glasses'. You only need the title if you aren't myopic.

Galloping myopia is what I have had since I was a child. Isn't it interesting the way a word commonly used in conjunction with another word conjures a kind of romance where otherwise there would be none? Galloping makes me think of horses. Stallions roaming wild and free. Extraordinary landscapes blurring into beauty.

Eyes failing to darkness because of galloping myopia – I struggle to find the beauty in that.

There were a series of horrible brown frames, which my mother then 'touched up' with pink nail polish. Galloping myopia meant the ophthalmologist recommended contact lenses for me. No Hollywood transformation here. Picture me, small and determined not to squint or squeeze my eyes shut against the certain invasion by a round, hard disc. I became extremely handy with gas permeable lenses; my only real anxiety was their displacement. During the monsoon, for example, when umbrellas were whipped out and crowds of parents, children and ayahs were whirling around each other, hustling to enter the school premises, spokes would whisk a lens out of my eye. Picture me, desperately scrabbling around dust and flapping at puddles to find the missing lens. It was a grisly business at times, but contacts are a blissful disguise of myopia.

Invisible frailties. I became a master of disguises at a young age. It is only now, after countless operations and scar tissue, that I feel incapable of disguising my visual frailty. It is there for you to see when I miss steps, when I need your arm to guide me, when I can't read any of those tiny behind-the-counter café menus.

I want a new pair of eyes. A fresh pair, youthful and sparkling with vitality. Mine are utterly worn out.

In my mind, I try to retrace my steps to retrieve that moment in the past, which led to this moment of my present, and all the fearful moments that lie in my future. But how far back shall I go? My paternal grandmother Ruqaiya's eyes were weak. If only she hadn't had myopia. Her story is my story, but only in part. Myopia can be managed with glasses and magnifiers and holding letters close to your eyes. You will fumble about at times, and in childhood you will be made fun of. But you can balance this frailty with other strengths, and only those close to you will know the truth of your seeing.

When we were children, my father used to draw his armchair up close to the television screen to watch cricket. It was normal. It never stopped him cheering more loudly than anyone else, roaring at a hoped for *six*! We found it comical the way he would roar equally loudly, but this time in distress, if any of us approached his eyes. We had no frame of understanding that many years earlier, he had lost his sight temporarily due to retinal detachments. One day, he had woken up unable to move or see. Paralysed and terrified, he mouthed the name of a fellow consultant at the Breach Candy Hospital.

Dr. Mehrani brought the antidote with him. He had suspected a calcium deficit, and injected Dad with calcium. Although Dad regained the ability to move, it was clear he needed eye operations. For six weeks he lay on a hospital bed, both eyes bandaged, while Mum read Louis L'Amour novels to him, worried about feeding her first born, three-month old son, because her breast milk had dried up from the trauma. From then on, both our parents lived in near permanent, but well-disguised fear of Dad losing his sight again. It took twenty-six years for that fear to manifest into reality.

My twin nieces have play scissors that they wield dangerously close to my eyes because they are being hairdressers and I need neatening up. A turn of my head and the scissor slices under my eyeball. I always try to temper my response so I don't frighten the girls and I don't burst into a storm of tears like they would, but I am afraid of those toy scissors in much the same way Dad would have been. Throughout my visual traumas, Dad has always maintained that our cases are different. That I must not look to his eventual blindness as the arc of my own story. I recognise the inherent kindness in his advice to disassociate my eyes from his, but fear pays little heed to kindness. A complex twenty-year case of steroid induced glaucoma, optic nerve damage and scar tissue formed around multiple eye operations, has left me in daily discomfort, but when I am asked a question as simply and clearly phrased as 'How are your eyes?' I have no ability to answer clearly or simply. Twenty years of ongoing visual trauma lends a fumbling quality to my response.

This is problematic in a doctor's room, where I am asked the exact same question, word for word. 'How are your eyes?' You might think I would stumble less, that the formal atmosphere of the Ophthalmology clinic might lend me fluency of jargon. But faced with the same question, and the same twenty-year history, I find myself just as deficient. I want time. I want a piece of paper and a pen. I want to write you an essay. Wait for me. I will find the right words. Just give me time.

Unlike myopia, which is a dull topic for the sighted, people are fascinated by degrees of blindness. Of ranges of visibility. If I mention my father is blind, the response is rarely one of immediate concern or pity. That is the second response. The first is always this: 'Is he completely blind? How much can he see? Some light? Anything?' Blind doesn't seem to convey the necessary impact. The audience in receipt of this bare fact seems always to be in need of comfort. I cannot provide comfort. He cannot see light.

My life with lupus often provokes a similar response in others: the desire to be comforted. By me. The sufferer.

'But, I mean, you can still live a normal life, right? It's not as though you are defined by the illness?'

A normal life? How? I am defined by this illness because there is no portion of me it has not touched.

How much can I see? is the wrong question to ask. How much I can see depends entirely on whether I am wearing contact lenses or not. That is the shared experience of myopia. We are thankfully living in a time when myopia (and most visual discrepancies) can be corrected by a pair of glasses, contact lenses or even, if you are so fortunate, successful laser surgery.

The real question is not *how much* can you see, but *how do* you see?

How do I see?
Sometimes, through a veil.

Imagine a chiffon scarf embroidered with scattered yellow dots. Lightning jags the centre and edges. It ripples. The lightning has a technical name: scintillating scotomas. They begin as spots of flickering lights, which devour my visual field in shimmering arcs or *teichopsia*, Greek for 'town hall' because they imitate the zigzagging patterns of fortified walls. The first time the fireworks in my eyes occurred, my nephew Rafael was about to be baptized; I was in church, and all I could do was hold on to my chair and trust that I would see again.

'Don't look at the light,' suggests Dr. Meyer, my medical ophthalmologist. As well tell me, 'don't breathe'. How can I survive without looking at light, looking for light?

The scotomas are temporary events. They pass, and I am left with a migraine. Is this a neurological condition? Is it vascular? Or simply rotten luck? Living with visual impairment is real. It is not in my head. But I live in my head, as we all do, as much as I live in my body. My eyes are what connect the two for the most part.

In September 2013, I had my third major eye surgery. The Molteno implant he had tucked into the upper left quadrant of my left eye, eight years earlier, was no longer functioning as powerfully as Keith, my surgeon, would like. He introduced a Baerveldt shunt in the only available space left by a trabeculectomy, a scleral graft and the implant. The new tube abuts my iris and rubs against my lens. I have been in ceaseless discomfort ever since. Something is rubbing constantly at my peace of mind. There is only so much ignoring you can do for visual discomfort, because most of our evasive techniques for pain are located in vision itself. Movies, books, walks in nature, cups of tea with a visiting friend, even lying in the dark, listening to music or a story. My eyes are click clacking to the sounds, blinking, blinking.

Only in sleep do I forget. Unless I dream the dreams of remembering.

There is one sightless comfort I can think of. Not being able to see people clearly or sometimes at all, can be very revealing. The true intent of a person is sometimes made clearer by the way they make me feel.

'One can never consent to creep when one feels an impulse to soar,' Helen Keller said. By the time she was seven, Keller was already in despair, not because she couldn't see or hear but because nothing had a name. And, she admits, she was spoiled rotten. Every plea for attention was rewarded by silencing her with sweets.

Then came Annie Sullivan.

And 'water' felt like it sounded, spilled into her hand. And 'doll' – the thing itself could be smashed against a wall – but the name? The name remained, carved, curled into the palm of her hand.

There are pictures of Helen dancing with Martha Graham, reading the lines of the faces of political heads like Ronald Reagan, Theodore Roosevelt and Jawaharlal Nehru, laughing with Alexander Graham Bell. Expecting the worst, she saw joy because the right person had entered her life and fought for her, advocating on her behalf until she had the language to do so herself. And on the birdwings of language she flew and flew into limitless skies.

To be a writer, you have to write. Words take time to form themselves. I am trying to write, trying to earn my place, but I struggle to keep faith when the words blur, when I lose my days to migraines. A few months ago, these migraines led to a vitreous detachment of my only functioning eye, and I am now beset by floaters, black cobwebs. I am never lost entirely to self-pity, but I do fear uselessness.

There is one anchor I use to keep myself afloat: in all the murk, I am able to determine colour. And this thought cheers me even as I swipe at the cobwebs and dervishes to keep still. A woman is standing by the newsagents in the hospital concourse. Her heels are neon orange. I want to rush up to her and thank her for the colour. I look down instead to write her into memory. When I look up again, she is gone. The fluorescent lights dotting the ceiling above the coffee shop's seating area await similar compliments, but they are no friends of mine. I have glaucoma. Hospital lighting creates a merciless environment for my eyes.

Prison, I think, would be worse.

But, one misery at a time, Shaista.

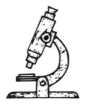

ON A SCALE OF ONE TO TEN

K eith often has a medical student in with him, or a visiting doctor from another hospital, another country.

This doctor is given access to my eyes in a way I can never access my eyes. 'Do you see the way the tube is sitting?' Keith asks. The student, or respected colleague, draws in a breath or makes no outward sound. It takes all my self-control to sit still, and act as though I am at ease with being viewed as object. This is science, I tell myself. Science.

Hospital is a place of work for everyone but the patient. As much as we may joke or even be serious about our lives with chronic illness resembling a full-time job, we know it isn't a job. At least not a recognisable one. Getting better as an occupation can only sound worthy on occasion. Every non-patient in hospital really does have a job, in the traditional sense, getting through their shifts, trying to do their best, making it to a break, and maybe punctuating the hours with banter. The hive is harmonious when you look at it from the outside, as you wait, post appointment, for a taxi. What a symphony the NHS is! What an orchestra!

Climb into the eye of the National Health Service, waiting for a follow up scan or procedure, and you become a number in a queue, jostling to be seen, to be heard, to be accounted for. And the paperwork that accumulates around you, threatens to erase the uniquely named human you thought you were.

⌒

I count the number of times I use the word 'pain' in a diary entry from my first year, post diagnosis. I find poetic devices to express everything but that word. After reading the earliest draft of my memoir, Caron Freeborn, a creative writing teacher on my MA programme, tells me I need to find a better alternative. 'The word pain loses meaning when repeated,' she says. I know exactly what she means. This does not make it any easier. I hold the Holy Grail in my hands: Helen McDonald's *H is for Hawk*. I want to meet Helen and shamelessly beg her for advice on how she wrote a book about grief without sprawling the word 'grief' on every page.

It's a crafty business figuring out your relationship with pain. On a scale of one to ten, how bad is your pain? In hospital, out of hospital, pain has to be scaled. Since the word is meaningless for anyone but the sufferer, it has to be measured cold. Looking into the eyes of your judge with her pen, notepad, questionnaire, you gauge for empathy, for humanity. Then you jump. Every number has a consequence. The trouble is you don't know which number equates to

a) nothing doing
b) Paracetamol
c) call the doctor for
d) something stronger.

You learn slowly.

A few years ago, I had a toenail infection. At first it looked like a little stain, a black line at the tip of my nail, probably too much nail polish application.

Then I showed it to my mother, which meant I was starting to get worried. Her response was quite breezy. Nails grow. Once it grows out, cut it.

I waited and waited. It was looking less than pretty. I went to the GP. We sent off nail clippings but because I was already on strong antibiotics for various other infections as well as immunosuppressive treatments, the findings were not sinister. I was prescribed nail lacquer. Months rolled by. One day, the pain.

Like when you catch your flesh in a door that slams shut on you. Or some small invisible tormentor is crushing bone and you can't hear it or see it, but you are sure it is the reason your toe is so swollen you can't bend it. Morning begins inside of the burning twisting nail and night falls on more of the same. To wear socks or not to wear socks.

You soak your toes in hot water and vinegar, then hot water and sea salt, then drown the digit in tea tree oil, Vicks vapo rub.

You remember from what seems like another lifetime, but was only the summer of 1998, a familiar excruciation when you had peripheral vasculitis and the splinter haemorrhages led to infection. Back then it was every single toe. You are grateful it is just one toe now. You lightly stroke the flesh of both feet, giving thanks for their years of being pretty and functional and infection free.

On a scale of one to ten, burn your scale. This pain belongs to the other scale, the one that begins

i) do you feel like you want to peel your nail off the bed,

ii) take a sponge drowned in candy floss scented ice numbing cool gel and

iii) swab the flesh until

iv) a new nail appears mid-air which you expertly slide back into your waiting flesh?

How do you keep sane when one organ, one digit, one ulcer is shrinking the attention of your brain to its epicentre? Enslaved, you rage.

Then change tactics and become very still. You have fibromyalgia, so you don't want the lines of trauma spreading, you don't want the talk of nails and explosions to rouse the sleeping Fibro Dragon. This must be contained at all costs.

You take a sleeping tablet. It doesn't work. How can it? There are little firecrackers letting themselves off in other parts of your body in preparation for a full-blown pain festival. I think about seeing a GP again. Hopefully not the same GP who tossed the nail lacquer at me, telling me this problem usually takes a year to clear up. I don't mind the year. I do mind the fire-breathing dragon living in my toe, preventing me from walking or sleeping.

I fantasise about meeting a GP who whips out a syringe filled with anaesthesia. 'Deep breath,' she says. I breathe in happy anticipation. She slides the needle in and I feel something cool and then nothingness. Before my eyes, I watch the transformation of bruised and infected to the kind of French polish glamour that used to be the fashion before nail art and bling.

I fantasise about healings. The cool water ripples of Reiki and the untangling of tangled symptoms through acupuncture. The bliss of a gentle massage is heavenly and the ease of a hot scented bath.

But instant healing, from a doctor?

My blackened toe grimaces at my naïveté. It knows I still long for such healing. It knows the best it can be given is the sense of gratitude learned from the nine toes that aren't assaulting my nerves, the ten fingers that are tapping away at creating sentences.

The Vietnamese Zen Buddhist monk Thich Nhât Hanh calls this type of practice Toothache Meditation. When you have a toothache, you think there is nothing more cruel. You cannot escape it. You become the toothache. But, Thây asks, what about all the days when you didn't have a toothache? We never even notice them. Toothache Meditation is for the days of no toothache – Dear Teeth, thank you for working well today, with no ache.

But I cannot be diligent all the time. The greatest pleasure of good health is the sheer effrontery with which we take every inch of our bodies for granted. Need to run for a bus? Your legs and arms will pump you there in time. Need to lift and carry heavy bags? Your back muscles and biceps will support you. Need to think, remember, study, excel? Your brain works wonders. Need to breathe? Here are your lungs. Here is your heart. Everywhere is your skin. And yet here we are, on the outside of our skin, looking in, wishing for something else. Invincibility. Magic wands.

The lupus body is one of the most tiring and vexing bodies of all. There are no limits to the inventiveness of such a disease. There is mercy shown – one organ or symptom that was critically in need may now appear stronger and self-able. But lo, just as you were contemplating a holiday abroad, a new degree, a spate of social engagements, the markers of your bloodwork start to trace mysteries of their own. Iron and magnesium too low. ESR too high. Cells are haemolising. Tissue is necrotising. You are falling to pieces again, and the shape of things to come is ugly and broken once more.

Nowadays, I struggle with the sound of the dawn parade of bird-song. It has heralded too many nights of endurance. Craters in my mouth. Migraines dancing across my skull. Muscle spasms. Belly cramps.

On a scale of one to ten, how do you bear it? You don't. The clock bears it for you.

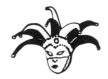

BUT YOU DON'T LOOK SICK

E ven when I do scale my pain accurately, there is still my unaccountably normal looking face to contend with.

There is gratitude in this. Society has never been kind to the Lucy Grealys of the world. A Ewing's sarcoma, and thirty years of reconstructive surgeries left poet and memoirist, Lucy Grealy, with facial disfigurements that made the mirror both her nemesis and fount of truth. Grealy wanted the autobiography of her face to match the beauty of her literary gifts. To match truth to beauty. After the publication of her memoir, Grealy believed she had made a contribution to society's seeming inability to see past outer disenchantments to inner enchantments. But a lifetime of depression and a heroin addiction led to her suicide. Wit carried her only so far. She didn't want to be the funny one. She wanted to be the beautiful one. She wanted to be herself, and not herself. She saw it all, saw through it all, and in the end, wanted neither illusion nor disillusion.

Sometimes at my worst, I'll try my best. I'll put on the Ritz.

Family friends will be visiting. Will have arrived at 10am or 12:30pm, and at 2pm, my body is still clinging to bed. Each minute, each quarter of the hour, I try to muster the necessary fuel to get going, and finally, I do it. Legs over the side, grip onto an imaginary rope and pull up. Change clothes. Brush hair. Laura Mercier the heck out of my dark circles. Then, I look kind of cute. And I start thinking, too cute! This is why people think you look really well!

Take the boots off and tone it down a notch. Standing in my socks changes everything. I shrink, for a start.

Wipe that bright lipstick off and go with the smudged lip balm effect.

Ok, better. Now they won't be befuddled by first being told 'Shaista isn't doing very well today', combined with me appearing like I'm about to 'do TV'.

The alternative – rolling down in my pyjamas – would embarrass my mother, who generally tries to hold her tongue on the state of my hair or appearance. Until or unless she can't. Modern sleepwear can, at a push, look somewhat casual cool. Black yoga pants. A soft cheerful sweatshirt. It can work. If it's accessorised with a smile. Rolling down in pyjamas and the mask of despair would probably try even my nieces and nephew. They aren't entirely without their own critiques. Eva, at four, comments on my pyjama clad state. 'But Shaista, why are you still in your pyjamas all day long?' She also comments on my messy room. Luckily, not my hair.

Once, standing in the kitchen, washing up with a friend, I talked about depression. The subject matter had been brought up by her, so I engaged. But perhaps too readily? Too fervently. Yes! Let's talk about depression! After a few minutes, she said, 'All this talk about depression has made me depressed.' I provided the expected sheepish grin, she sidled away.

With almost every social encounter, I get asked, 'How are you?' A perfectly valid question. A perfect zinger for a human with an A4 length page of co-morbidities.

When you ask me how I am, or even how I am *today* (nice and specific), I generally go into brain melt down, Pollock style. I am sifting through my body. You are not my Rheumatology or Immunology consultant, but you care about my health. I want to gift you the right answer but which one? How are *you* feeling today? Which answer can *you* handle? And all the while we both know no matter what I say, whichever route I take – through wit or despair – we will return to 'But You Don't Look Sick!'

It's all a game. The well person engages the sick person in the game of 'Let's Pretend' by saying, 'But you don't look sick'. Then it is up to the sick person to either bat back a light-hearted comment, thereby playing the game, or end the game by introducing the spectre of mortality: *I may look well, but I am sick. You could get sick too. We are all going to die.* Ghoulish, but true.

No chronically sick person can avoid the suspicion of being considered a toxic body by the healthy observer. Possibly contagious. 'Get well!' instruct their cards. As though you were, in fact, aiming to do the opposite. You were hoping to 'Stay Sick!' But now you might consider their positive adjuration. Behind the word 'But' (which is what makes the sentence problematic), is this idea: 'Since you don't look sick, have you considered the possibility that you might not *be* sick? I'm just putting it out there. Think about it.'

Society's questions and comments are mirrored by my doctors. *How are you? You look well! Are you feeling better now? What have you been up to?* My answers have no real consequences outside the doctor's clinic. Inside, the consequences, always unknown, can be life changing.

There is a slippery, sliding scale of how I am, how anybody with chronic illness is. The failure on our part to accurately describe, define and thereby deal with our particular illness lends inauthenticity to our narrative. If we really knew what was wrong, we would be able to fix it. So perhaps the fact that we don't know as much as others feel we should, indicates the possibility that we are fake or phony. That the illness is imaginary. Psychosomatic. Hysterical. All in our head.

There is a certain infamy to being ill. If the diagnosis is cancer, there is the cachet of mortal danger. If it is auto-immunity, there is the uniqueness of your position in the lives of family and friends. You are often the only one in your circle with this dragging at the heels of your life. And the conundrum everyone faces is this: support you as you are or try to fix you. Love is helpful. Love is kind. Love is concerned. But love is also busy attending to other loves and other needs. In the stretches of time between offerings of support or help, a person with chronic illness must get on with herself. Days, weeks, sometimes months of an isolation that is not necessarily the most brutal thing. An ill-judged comment can undo weeks of lovely self-acceptance.

When I was holed up on the Rheumatology ward the summer before I turned twenty, bright glorious days of sunshine flooded in and every morning the nurses would draw the blinds. Mostly out of routine and habit, but also to enjoy the seasonal warmth. I was suffering from intense photophobia, burying my face in my pillows to block out the light. I had not yet been diagnosed with glaucoma or retinal vasculitis. My mother suggested sunglasses. It was embarrassing, but since I couldn't keep leaping out of bed to draw back the blinds, it was a solution of sorts. When I was moved into a room of my own, I relaxed into an illusion of privacy. One afternoon, a health care assistant about my age, walked in, and seeing my sunglasses, asked me who I thought I was: a celebrity? Or did I think I was at the beach?

When she left, my flood of tears startled everyone in the room.

I was checked on constantly, so word of my outburst reached the senior staff nurse and I never saw the young health care assistant again.

Over the years, I have re-lived this moment in my mind, re-examining the lines of context. I have been the youngest person on the ward for many years, being tended to by equally young or even younger nurses. The instinctual perception that had me cringing at the idea of wearing sunglasses indoors was the knowledge that although our peers may be the least sensitive, they are also necessary mirrors of ourselves. Of our possible selves. That young health care assistant may have been trying to connect with possibly the only young patient on the ward. Maybe she was trying to make me laugh. It is unlikely she was being deliberately provocative, deliberately unkind. But she was not skilful in her care.

Just as non-patients lack the innate verbal skills that would most wisely and compassionately suit a patient, so patients lack the necessary skill in dealing with the healthy world. And we are far more invested in not alienating our peers with clumsy responses. There is no subtlety to their thought processes at play. If you are young, why are you on a ward in hospital? Why aren't you out in the real world, being young? What is really being asked is this: why aren't you more like me?

In his book *The End of Your Life Book Club*, Schwalbe references *The Etiquette of Illness* by Susan Halpern, a cancer survivor. The subtitle of Halpern's book is 'What To Say When You Can't Find The Words'. Written in 2004, it was seven years too late for freshly diagnosed eighteen-year-old me, who was desperate for such a book. Here is a piece paraphrased by Schwalbe that might have saved me great mental anguish:

Halpern wants the reader to think about the difference between asking 'How are you feeling?' and 'Do you want me to ask how you're feeling?' Even if it's your mother whom you're questioning, the first approach is more intrusive, insistent, demanding. The second is much gentler and allows the person simply to say no on those days when she's doing well and doesn't want to be the 'sick person', or is doing badly but wants a distraction, or has simply been asked the question too many times that day to want to answer it again.

My book could as easily be titled *The Etiquette of Illness* because I have been in pursuit of understanding the etiquette of illness ever since I was diagnosed. Healing is a fragile business. There is only so much 'help' one can look for, outside of the self, in books and advice and the wisdom of others. The only true healing I have ever experienced has come with time and a gentleness fostered by patient loving kindness towards myself, and the patient loving kindness of my parents. Healing and slowness maintain a deep partnership in my life but understanding the significance of slowness in the first years of the lupus miasma was painful for me. As were the many offerings of 'you can heal yourself if you just do/don't do…' that still proliferate.

One of my truths is this: if I could stay silent, I would. But I can't. Partly because the world — the smaller world that cares about me — won't allow it. And partly because I am a writer. I am in a relentless relationship with words. Words that separate me from harmony and wholeness, and words that connect me. Connect us.

It isn't always easy to connect. The telephone has long heralded its own form of torture. Of course, the social majority now doesn't engage with live telephone calls anyway. It has become a running joke that if you message someone and they respond with an actual phone call, you drop the phone in horror. What are they doing calling you?! You were probably in the bathroom, maybe in the bath. Or still in bed with sleep hair and sleep eyes. With the addition of the video option, our filter of privacy is even easier to disrupt.

But I have older echoes of anxiety. Every time the phone rings, I have to steel myself for, 'How are you? Still sick? Why?' The same call and response throbs as you wait outside a doctor's office. You know you'll be asked this question and you have to prepare your defence.

Why are you here? With 'here' meaning 'in hospital' for a doctor and 'in bed/ at home/ not working' for a friend or relative. For a doctor, your defence involves trying to justify how ill you are, and for a non-medic, it involves having to play it down. The contortions involved in distinguishing between modes of communication are exhausting.

Here are the three options for a sick person:
1) Get Better.
2) Die Trying.
3) Write A Book. (Preferably a cookbook. One out of six books on the New York Times health bestseller list is food or diet related.)

I was a good student at school. Obedient. Embarrassed to step out of line and be punished. Punishment always seems such a public display. A performance in itself. I was a teenager when I was diagnosed and a part of me still responds to both the medical institution and social attitudes towards illness much as I did at school.

What would disobedience entail here? Have I ever been disobedient? Yes, inherently so. I am not getting better. The code of sick to better that informs the outside world also informs the inside world of hospitals. After all, the work of a doctor is to heal you. You are the dysfunctional material that must be wrought to function better. Ideally to function perfectly. The fiction involved in that language is never more clearly displayed than in the case of a lupus patient. It is not that we cannot get better, but that we are still so far from being understood. We are functioning imperfectly and chaotically because of an authority more powerful than any doctor. We contain a universe of anti-double stranded DNA. We produce immune complexes whose peculiar formations the medical world is still trying to perceive let alone successfully unravel.

Part of 'But you don't look sick/ At least you look really well' is the sound of the outer world almost sighing with relief. A voiced gratitude that the illness may have come but it hasn't conquered what matters, which isn't necessarily outer beauty, but that the person you love still looks like the person you loved. Since we associate illness with death, we fear that illness will begin its theft by taking away pieces of the outer body. Hair, apple cheeks, limbs. When we see that nothing has been lost visually, we cannot help but proclaim, 'I counted and it's all there. You don't look sick. Whew!'

Doctors have said, 'You look well!' to me time and again over the years and when these same doctors have come to care for me, I can no longer consider this comment thoughtless or alienating. They are relieved and cannot hide their relief.

It is counter-productive for me, the patient, who now has to drag the conversation back to less uplifting tones. And this tricky back pedalling from nicety to social unpleasantness is why the comment is almost impossible to navigate. Often, doctors may catch themselves, 'I know you probably don't feel as well as you look...' which offers the patient the chance to leap in with, 'I don't!' but you still feel like the ungrateful person on Christmas morning, who is glad there was a gift but wished it contained what you wanted rather than what you were given. Compliments feel this way to a chronically sick person. You want them, you need them. You prefer them to 'You look really tired today. Your eyes are so blood shot!' You just wish they wouldn't arrive at quite the moment they do. Before you have had a chance to say *my insides don't match my outside, so please, go gently with me today*. Looking well, equals being well, strong, healthy, confident. It also implies a normalcy has been attained.

A compliment that I would gladly receive would be an acknowledgement on the part of my observer that somehow, despite the years of illness theft – and there have been thefts, whether you can see them or not – I still hold up. I can still present myself in a manner that does not entirely displease my mother. Between you and me, she is the only one from whom I really need to hear the words, 'You are beautiful, my daughter.'

When someone compliments me on my looks, on looking well, I fill in the blank with 'for a sick person'. I take that as the precise compliment. If, after twenty years of illness and cytotoxic medications, I still look good to you, then I'll just go ahead and brush my shoulders off, because that is something to be glad about, something I don't take for granted. I know how easily this disease can rob me of my senses, my organs, my limbs, my functions.

The difference between receiving the compliment in my first years and now, is that I know, and maybe you know now, the life-threatening nature of this disease. We didn't know it then. We couldn't know it then. So, when you praised me, it sounded like you were brushing my illness away. You couldn't see it, so it didn't exist. When you acknowledge another human being's suffering, you see them, you really see them. After that, you can compliment them all you like. In the context of understanding one another, compliments become love poems, celebrations of each other's beauty. Celebration because we are both alive and it could so easily be otherwise.

Sometimes a point has to be reached when you stop saying to a sick person, 'Yes, but... you can do better.' Instead, you simply listen, and then say, 'I understand.' Even if you don't. Even if the voice in your head is pounding out the words, 'Yes, but... Don't give up! You can do this! Be positive! You never know!'

Sometimes you need to recognise when a person needs to be seen as they truly are, in that moment of despair without your desperate, flailing attempts to glue them back together with encouragement and cheerleading. We all need encouragement and good cheer, but the chronically ill patient is rarely allowed even a nanosecond to be her real self. Light will filter through, eventually, regardless of your pep talk.

What we are often craving is to be allowed to be seen broken, mask off, and still be loved.

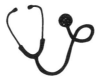

THE ART OF ASKING (FOR LOVE)

Here is a good description of the pathogenesis of lupus:

The disease is an immunologic disorder marked by the presence of circulating immune complexes. Active disease is associated with raised circulating immune complexes and reduced fractions of complement.

Diagnostic tests: anti DNA antibodies, mitochondrial type V antibodies.

I copied the above into my 2005 journal from a textbook titled *Clinical Ophthalmology* by Jack J. Kanski, while I was an in-patient on the Eye Unit, awaiting the Molteno tube implant and the transplant of a scleral graft. I spent part of my sluggish hours drawing pictures of artificial filtering shunts and teaching myself about aqueous outflow and sub-Tenon's space. I can carefully introduce medical jargon here about auto-antibodies, T cells and B cells, but I could never use these terms authoritatively or casually, like Kanski can.

Sometimes a doctor will refer to the effects of a drug or the inevitability of a certain symptom the way an English teacher might refer to the rule of capitalizing the first letter of a sentence: obvious, common knowledge. Excuse me, I want to point out, I've been on the drug for years and no one ever mentioned this nugget of information.

Lab tests. Lab rats. We are lab rats with no education. Doctors, with all their knowledge, impart nothing to us of understanding the microbial, immunologic structure behind the outer face of lupus. We, patients, learn little that is medically related at school. We are intensely ignorant when we walk through a doctor's door and into their safe place. The hospital has been their home for many years; even if you're both newbies, you're also on the wrong side to be friends.

Here is another quote that makes more sense to me, from Amanda Palmer's *The Art of Asking*:

> *And so often, underneath it all, these questions originate in our basic human longing to know: Do you love me?*
> *How do we ask each other for help? When can we ask? Who's allowed to ask?*

'Do you love me?' This simple, impossible question lives at the heart of my daily quest. It is my quest in ordinary life, so how can it cease to be relevant when I enter the hospital domain? It becomes more relevant than ever. Love is the unmentionable word in hospitals. A patient must not love her doctor – that is dangerous. Have you heard of a doctor loving a patient who is not a family member or friend? Is it even allowed? Am I allowed to ask? I'm asking.

In *The Art of Asking*, Palmer stresses that the shame and embarrassment that accompany the artist who asks for help is counterproductive. Working artists and their supporting audiences are two necessary parts in a complex ecosystem. Palmer's explanation of the relationship between art and audience mirrors how I feel about medicine, and the complex ecosystem in which the medic and the patient exist. It is an incredibly imbalanced system. The power lies almost entirely with everyone who isn't the patient. We, patients, are helpless, clueless and in pain. We are frightened and not only do we not have the language necessary to understand the answers, we do not possess the language necessary to ask the right questions. We talk in riddles. In childish phrases.

It hurts. Here.

Can you be more specific? On a scale of one to ten?

No, I can't be more specific. It. Just. Hurts.

I am the daughter of a doctor. I have something of an 'in' with medi-speak. When I stumble on terms and technology, I ask my father for help. And even with his knowledge and guidance, I have been, I am, endlessly vulnerable.

My local GP clinic is full of decent folk, doing their best, generally well liked in the village. But even after twenty years of clinic visits, I have made no friends among the local medics. I was an outsider when I arrived because of my race and I continue to be an outsider now because I have a disease that is not welcome. A recently retired GP at our practice made this comment: 'If you have a non-lupus related, non-immunology based problem, you are welcome to come and see me. If it's lupus, don't come.'

I have Systemic Lupus Erythematosus. Emphasis on *systemic*. This is a disease that affects every part of my body in insidious ways that are invariably lupus related. What problem could my body possibly throw up that can't be traced back to lupus?

My GP didn't want to be the middleman between the hospital and me. He considered himself an honest man. It was his trademark. But while I attempted to respect his honesty, I was simultaneously holding back the waters of a memory well full of tears. Lupus is not loved. Is any disease loved by doctors? I circle back: do doctors love patients? Patients sometimes love doctors. There seems to be only a one-way flow of love and even this is just as easily revoked when a patient feels threatened or neglected.

Is love not possible here?

It is a bleak conclusion to draw, but one that is supported by Jerome K. Groopman in his book *How Doctors Think*. Chronically sick patients are the least liked by doctors because of feelings of failure when dealing with diseases that resist therapy. I had only a suspicion this was true. Now there is written proof.

To be a patient is to be aware of the fraught tension between being a human in need of healing, and a body being experimented upon. We are privy to cases of power abuse in fiction – Victor Frankenstein – and in real lives – Einar Wegener and Alan Turing. Gendered abuse, under the sweeping diagnosis of hysteria, by male doctors upon the female bodies in their care, is still rife.

During a three-month admission in 2009, when my symptom of lymphedema was as yet uncontrolled, a consultant told me in graphic detail about one of his female patients whose bladder functionality was disturbed, as mine appeared to be. She had adjusted well to diapers, this consultant shared, offering me what he considered a plausible solution. I can still picture myself looking up at him from my shrunken position on the bed, as he casually tossed me a future, using another woman's suffering as anecdote. I felt her pain, her discomfort, her shame, even though he gave her no name, no identity beyond an animal body. A code was being broken in the sharing of this story, but in a manner too nuanced for me to denounce.

Once, when a urinary tract infection stubbornly resisted the first course of antibiotics, I returned to my GP clinic. The doctor who had prescribed the first course had been mild-mannered, gentle and gentlemanly, perhaps even old-fashioned, speedily concluding his assessment because there was nothing complicated about either diagnosis or deliverance. The second doctor introduced me to a new experience. He was a locum I had never met before. I explained I had a UTI that hadn't been resolved. He wanted to know if I was a nurse or a medic. *Why?* I asked. Because UTI was medical jargon, and how else would I have access to such knowledge? I explained further that I had systemic lupus, a long-term illness, so shortening words to acronyms was hardly beyond my remit as patient. He became technical. He wanted to know the details of my personal life. Was I married or did I have a boyfriend? I said I had neither. He was shocked. How could that be? At this point, I found myself looking around for a hidden camera. When he began asking me my techniques for self-hygiene, in which direction I washed myself, I was sure I had fallen into a surrealist play, only I didn't know my lines, and I felt profoundly unsafe. When I left his office, I was in a daze. At home, I recounted the incident to my mother, who thought I should make a complaint to the manager of the clinic, but at that moment a friend of mine rang. His take was humorous: a failed flirtation was his perception of the incident. I began to wonder if I had over-reacted. And, simultaneously, that I couldn't bear the thought of recounting the incident again and again to the other predominantly male GPs at the clinic. If my friend's reaction was typical, then I would appear unnecessarily thin-skinned. The shame, suffice to say, was all mine.

For most of my life, I have suffered the various ignominies of heavy periods, and during one of several admissions on the Infectious Diseases ward, bleeding alarmingly, fibroids were flagged on an abdominal CT scan. A gynaecologist visited me. She had a young, vibrant energy to her. She must have already seen my age on my notes, because she burst in with a series of pre-formed questions. Did I have children? Did I want children? If I didn't, she could simply burn my womb. Words like hysterectomy and cauterisation punched out of her. She wanted to know when I had last had sex. I spoke quietly and quickly, sharing things I'd never shared with a doctor before, hoping my words would not find their way into notes shared publicly on the e-hospital system, but needing to say them, come what may.

India is home to a billion people and seems to house the entire range of humanity and inhumanity. In a country heaving with aimless, wandering male youths, the violation of the female body is commonplace. Walking to school, men would brush past me, their fingers taking full advantage of pavement proximities in a coordinated assault. My mother's decision to have an ayah accompany me to and from school didn't dissuade the predators because my ayah was a woman too. Home also ceased to be a sanctuary because we had live-in male domestic staff, common in Indian households. One day, when I was eight or nine years old, leaning against the protective wooden sideboard of my bed, immersed in my book, I didn't notice until our seventy-year old, stately, duster of the house, was standing behind me, cupping the small bumps on my chest. He made a comment in Hindi about how much I had grown, that I was not a little girl anymore. I froze until he moved away. Later, in my first romantic relationship, this frozen movement, still buried in memory, made every act of intimacy feel like an assault. Evading consummation eventually resulted in the ultimate betrayal on his part – my repeated, whimpered *no* was ignored, and I became that othered thing, victim to the oldest theft. It happened long ago, and I have let no one touch me since.

On a bed in a hospital ward, our secret selves are forced to reveal themselves.

Why do I share this in a book about chronic illness? I place the parallel tale of my body here, so you understand that for the girl woman boy man who must lie, naked and vulnerable before the doctor's penetrating gaze and educated touch, an echoing heartbeat of fear accompanies every examination. It is not anxiety. It is the memory of knowing. It is precaution. It does not have to be told, but spoken or unspoken, it is part of who I am. I have not escaped its legacy.

The quality of my gynaecologist's listening had been absolute and acute. She softened, and gentled, and rubbed my knee. She apologised. A general apology for the state of the world in which such things happen. I was grateful for her kindness, at the end, but not her initial abrasions.

⁓

Waiting outside a clinic for a doctor we may or may not have met before, our anxiety peaks. Even if we have met the doctor before, several times perhaps, we are still going to be meeting them for the first time that day, that hour. Which facet of the doctor will we see today? Impossible to predict. I have lost count of the number of times I have been advised to wear a thick skin upon entering the doctor's office, by my father, by solicitous friends. It seems to me an extraordinary expectation to demand of a human being who is at her most thin-skinned, literally naked, if she is undergoing a physical examination. Thick skins are for the outside world of strangers, and even then, I have always struggled with knowing when to don and when to remove skins.

Some years ago, I was hoping to change my mobile phone contract to a pay as you go. It had been a mistake to sign up for a contract but negotiating with the salesman on the phone, when in the throes of a feverish flare, had led me into the sticky trap. At the mobile phone store in town, another salesman, far from being more compassionate when face to face with a fellow human, became more specifically cruel. 'Even if you were dying,' he said, 'you wouldn't be able to get out of your contract. You would have to actually die.' I remember wondering if I ought to tell him I had cancer. I knew I couldn't tell him I had lupus. He wouldn't have heard of it. It would have meant nothing. Would cancer have moved him? But he had already dismissed the prospect of me dying.

People often like to tell me about the 'real world', which they presume doesn't penetrate the sick person's bubble. It is quite the opposite. The sick person is more porous than most. We may try not to focus on our minor shames, humiliations and lamentations, but these constitute the precise reason a human being with a name and a destiny struggles with being a number in a bureaucratic system.

E-hospital 'went live' a few years ago. Computerised data is aiming to make life easier for medical staff but the patient was never consulted in this re-haul. My data from the very first day I set foot on National Health Service soil, which lived for years in notes gathering dust and curled edges, is now accessible to any NHS staff member; I am the only person who cannot easily access my data. I, the body itself, the home of the cells, move further and further away from what the doctor sees. Does modern data access make modern doctors feel more secure? Do medics feel safer being able to rely on facts, figures and scales of pain? Hippocrates and Galen would be appalled. In spite of my vulnerability, I find myself requesting doctors to listen to my chest, my pulse. Look at me, really look at me, I want to say. I, the patient body, am here for you to look at. But the modern patient often looks too well for doctors to rely on the body anymore.

'Barcodes. We are barcodes,' says a woman on my left, in the infusion bay. 'It's dehumanising.'

'Like you're products!' chimes in the nurse, who is scanning her into a computer.

Words used neatly are gifts we patients give each other. Later, across the room, I will hear another patient joke about barcodes.

It never gets easier.

It's a bit like school; you went there every day for years without end in sight, but you never strolled in, utterly confident and expectant, knowing exactly what and where your place was. There were always nerves because there were teachers, figures of authority who could dole out punishment or praise. You were never privy to their machinations.

When I walk into hospital, I experience a similar combination of anxiety and belonging. I never know if I'll get told off or comforted. I try to be myself but that's not much good because inevitably, in an institution as colossal as the NHS, the individual is an unwelcome intrusion. So I try with various ounces of energy to make hospital habitable. I engage my fellow human beings in social conversation, exchange seeming commonplaces, make points of contact.

In the hospital concourse, at the M&S checkout till, I tell the tiller my name. I introduce myself this way: 'I'm Shai.' And then, when he bats back: 'You don't seem shy!' I produce my full name, phonetically. Shy Star. There is something curiously intimate about a stranger sounding out your name. He says it so loudly I almost regret the personal touch. Almost, but not enough. No matter how many times I decide I cannot, will not expose myself to further vulnerabilities in this soul-stealing building, I always, always try to connect. It's a curse as much as a blessing.

On a day when I have a brain scan, I walk to the wrong department, unknowingly. The nurse at the MRI desk asks another staff member for help in finding my name on the computer. Together they locate me, but I am in the wrong scanning department. Apparently, there are several. One of the women tells me she will direct me to the right department. I thank her and follow her out. Turns out it is MRIS I need, not MRI.

'What does the 'S' stand for?' I ask. 'Scan?'

'Spectroscopy, I think,' she says, and then, when I make another comment in response to hers: 'Can I just direct you, please?'

'Yes, of course,' I say, hiding my embarrassment.

After I've walked in the direction she pointed out, I stand leaning against a wall for a few seconds, fighting back tears. Over the next few minutes, I watch nurses direct people to various parts of the hospital. Their exchanges are friendly. No tears shed (that I can see).

I am about to have a brain scan. I appreciate that this is a normal day's work and therefore my guide felt no hesitation in conveying how important her time was and how I was wasting precious seconds of it with my idle chatter. But it wasn't really idle chatter. I genuinely wanted to know the difference between MRIS and MRI, because I was about to have one of them and not the other.

You need a thicker skin, I've been told a thousand times.

In this place, how? This is the place I have to bare my skin, volunteer my cells, blood, marrow, and soon, prepare my skull for examination.

My mother had dropped me off because parking at the hospital is difficult. I should have asked her to stay. She would have found a way if I had made it clear I wanted her, needed her, to stay. But you never know which day will be the one filled with kindness and which day will decimate you with the tiniest cruelty. I try to be independent, to navigate these corridors on my own. I've navigated them since I was eighteen. That should count for something. But it counts for very little.

You need to learn to say NO. Speak your mind. Speak UP! I've been told a thousand times.

I am not a perfect candidate for anything other than being the smiling one. I over-smile. I over-share. This is a thing these days. Over-sharing. It means you have made others uncomfortable. You know they are uncomfortable because they become unkind.

I like smiling. It makes me happy. I smile at the patient being wheeled by in her bed. She doesn't smile back. I smile at the group of hijabis who walk past me like black lotuses floating across the cement. One smiles at me. Yes! I low five myself.

In the end, I don't have the brain scan. The radiographer is uncomfortable with the idea of my Baerveldt shunt. He has never heard of such a device in all his years of medicine. I explain it was an operation to control glaucoma. I even give him a little peek into my eye. But I happily agree with his considered opinion that we postpone the brain scan until he has investigated the mechanism of a Baerveldt shunt. I feel sure my brain is fine. And even if there is some inflammatory cerebral lupus activity, what treatment can I possibly have for it that I haven't already been prescribed?

While I am sitting in the waiting room, I think about my last brain scan, some years ago. I wrote about it on my blog and compared my experience to the experience of the children of Gaza. Not to be perverse – because obviously there is no actual comparison – but I was trying to imagine, while I lay inside the deafening tunnel, what it must be like for a child with shrapnel in her skull, undergoing MRI scans (if she can get to a decent hospital). Doubly horrific, I thought, to lie there, body constricted, sounds like gunfire exploding around your head.

There is a kind of violence we experience in hospital. '*You're just running all over the hospital, aren't you?*' one of my first consultants barked at me. The level of intimidation he imposed, instilled in me a deep-seated fear of the power doctors can wield, the violence that can be inflicted by words.

We are without boundaries in here. We are organs and blood, lymph and nerve. And we are facing suits with rulebooks we were not handed. This is a place of terror. You leave your human self outside the doors, and enter, naked and shaking. Your life is about to change. Nodules may be found. Tumours. Or nothing. You may be pronounced normal. And your mind falls under suspicion of imagining things. Either way you are damned. People walk purposefully down these corridors only when they are not the damned. Twenty years later, I have indeed 'run all over the hospital'. Ghosts of memories, old selves, skin cells are gathered here.

Time is suspended in the waiting room. We are trapped.

These aren't my words. Someone skimmed them across the waiting room at the eye clinic one day; they were so perfectly formed, I intercepted them.

Your appointment time is just the beginning of your negotiation with time. Gathered into that suspended time is the amalgam of all our anxieties, our household burdens, our monetary woes. Very little is spoken out loud. It is all energy sensed, shared by osmosis.

My heart is a single man's marching band in tune with a phone ringing that nobody is picking up. There is always a phone ringing on the wards that nobody seems to want to pick up. Haven't we all been on the dialing end?

I see the lovely face of one of the kindest nurses. She mouths, *how are you?* I smile or shrug. One develops an interesting set of body language skills to convey social niceties in a place like this. And all the time, there is the thump-thump of nerves that accompany you as you wait for a sentence to be delivered. This is a court of law, and the consultant and registrar are your judge and lawyer. I wonder what it feels like to be on the other side, behind that closed door. There is no waiting on the other side; knowledge lies on the other side of that door. In the waiting room, we have only the energy of anxious ignorance, cloaking and paralysing us.

Even outside the door of my favourite doctor, Keith, who calls me 'old friend' before correcting himself (*sorry, less of the 'old', right?*), even outside his door, I can't decide which face to display. Shaista, who has a quick wit and wry sense of humour? Shaista, who is nine fathoms deep in depression and wants only to climb out of her skin, and in to new, fresh, surgery free flesh? Or the quiet Shaista, who can neither quip nor question, nor even cry? That is the Shaista he probably hopes never to see.

Shaista with the fire is always better than Shaista with no hope.

(BE) THE WARRIOR

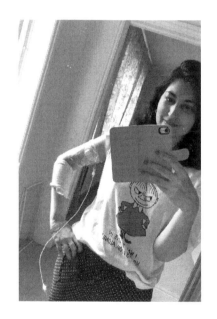

Exuberance

I have high fevers and night sweats.
My fingers and toes flush hot and cold

and transform
into purple flowers.

My face, that transient thing,
breaking up and taking shape,

a sweet moon
in a thunder cloud sky.

In moments of perfect beauty,
my face reveals its grace.

Lupus, you odd unnatural thing,
I am razing you to the ground.

Here, on the ward, I am laughing,
I am offering you my exuberant soul.

Take it,
if you dare.

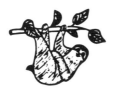

BED

Let me try telling it this way.

Draw a horizontal line. On one side write *life* and on the other, *death*. If you perceive life moving towards death in a chronological fashion, then you'll probably write *life* on the left and *death* on the right. Or you'll put *death* on the left and *life* on the right. Death as a beginning. Darkness as a beginning. Moving towards light, towards life.

Now collapse the centre point of your line into a sunken bowl.

This is chronic illness. Chronic illness is the in between place of stuck. Life shouts out to you, *grab hold of me! Come on, I'll pull you across with my words and these movies and this travel brochure.* Death says nothing. But life looks at you, knowingly. *Is that what you want? To just give up and die? Fight! This is the good side!* Life is the place where everything happens, from the expected to the unexpected; the learning to walk, run, drive, feel, study, make money, lose property and possessions, create more of yourself, grow. Death, they tell us, is the place where it ends. All the money, the property, the human bodies you loved but cannot pull across to the other side with you.

In between, in the place of stuck, we share the human terror of a life with no possible change. So deeply uncomfortable are we with the place where nothing seems to happen, that we plague each other by asking the question, 'What do you *do*?' What do you do with your life?

Not, who are you in your life? Not, how do you feel in your skin? Your mind? Your heart? But, where in the cogs do you fit?

An odd character with the wolf disease is bound to feel defensive about what she does, mostly because she doesn't. You would think that when I am in hospital, I would be let off this hook for a bit.

In 2017, I was hospitalised four times with persistent infections. It was a complex year to navigate. On two separate occasions, I had to have a PICC line: a slender catheter surgically inserted into my vein, one end hanging outside my skin, for me to self-administer liquid antibiotics, and the other end resting atop my heart. Self-administration makes me respect my nurses even more than usual; there are so many little details to concentrate on, air bubbles and contaminations to be careful of. On each occasion, I administered thirty-two infusions, some at home, and some at the hospital as an in-patient. Rheumatology suspected that my long-term monoclonal antibody therapy had resulted in my body becoming more immuno-compromised than ever. Immunology disagreed and pointed to my underlying hypergammaglobulinemia. Either way, the reality of such immunological machinations was a bone deep fatigue. I needed to rest.

And yet, I lost count of the number of times I was teased by medical staff about sleeping. Do other patients rise and shine, stretch and leap out of their narrow white beds to... do what?

'So,' asked my consultant when she visited, 'what have you been up to in here? Working on anything?'

'Working on getting this fever down,' I replied.

During my fourth admission of the year, I was moved from a ward on the ground floor (Gastrology) up to the tenth floor (Infectious Diseases), to an enclosed room, with negative pressure-controlled vents circulating eddies of freezing cold mechanical air. I was on heavy anti-biotics. Rizwan brought me blankets, a beanie hat and gloves the first night, because I could not stop shivering.

'Every time I've seen you,' said a male nurse the next day, 'you've been sleeping!'

'What should I be doing?' I asked. 'Inventing a new gadget?'

His comment stuck, and from then on, I fought sleep to occupy myself – painting in watercolour and pastel, writing blog posts, trying to look busy to account for the bizarre preoccupation of society even on the most isolated Infectious Diseases ward to *DO SOMETHING DO ANYTHING JUST DO SOMETHING!*

So, I did do something. Only it was accidental. I pushed open the heavy door to my room, stepped out, ostensibly to discover when my next antibiotic dose was, and had a quiet mooch down the long, unfamiliar corridor ahead of me. There are eleven beds on the Infectious Diseases ward, each locked away from the other. Towards the end of the corridor, I saw a portrait of Mary Seacole on the wall. *Hello, Mary*! I greeted it. I had reached the fire door now, and while contemplating Mary, I leant companionably against the door. Suddenly, a wild alarm set off, ringing around the ward. I put my hands up in true crime drama fashion as two burly male nurses hefted their way towards me. *Sorry!* I bleated, recognising one of them, and slunk away from the crime scene.

'You won't be doing that again,' he called out after me.

Honestly. Can't win. Back to bed I went.

During my 2005 admission on the Eye Unit, while undergoing various surgical procedures like needling and the laser-burning of ciliary bodies in the hope of bringing my intra-ocular pressures down, a friend visited. *Had I been down to the concourse for a little shopping?* she asked. How could I blame her? I had done precisely that on the first day of my admission, whizzing about The Body Shop, buying presents for the Kawanos, Irfan's Japanese landlord and landlady, who were visiting England for the first time.

Try the Shepherd's pie! my friend advised, looking at my lunch menu.

I did. When my eye pressures shot up later that evening, and my oph-thalmologist, Dr. Meyer, found me violently retching up that same concoction, how could I blame my friend for her cheerful suggestion?

You are tired. *How is your mood?* the doctor will ask you. *You mean my mental health?* you wonder. I am tired. Fatigue is an actual symptom but mention it to a doctor and they will tell you to *try doing a little more every day. Try exercise. Try T'ai Chi.*

The inner persona of the professional bed resting human may con-fidently follow the motto of 'Just Do Nothing' as opposed to 'Just Do It', but our outer persona will always be subject to scrutiny. Doing nothing in the face of a busy, restless world, will never be met with anything other than baffled curiosity, at best. At worst, a thinly veiled contempt. *Have you ever tried waking up early?* they will ask. *Exercising last thing at night, to tire you out? Baths, to make you sleepy? Yoga? Going vegan?* Battleground language begins here. Get up. Escape. Be a (Wo)Man.

If only being tired were an Olympic sport, or the subject of a dis-sertation. Sleep is never enough. All sleep is forcibly ended with alarm clocks or guilt. The shock of waking never fails to unnerve me.

In my second year at university, I met a poet called Les Murray. Not the way I would later meet his contemporary, Clive James, across our portable motor pumps on the Patient Short Stay Unit, but on the page, in poetry. There were poems that could only have been created by an Australian bard writing within the Jindyworobak tradition, but there was one that spoke directly to me as though it had been written for me. One that I have carried with me all the years since. It is titled 'Homage to the Launching Place' and is just that. Each line pays homage to '*bed, kindest of quadrupeds*'.

'*I loved you from the first, bed/ doorway out of this world*', writes Murray, thereby giving me the line upon which I can hang my own love. Every time I climb back into my bed, and it is always 'back', a return home, I feel as though I am being welcomed, the way a beloved house greeted you, greets you still.

When we were children, my mother agreed to temporarily take care of a neighbour's golden retriever. He was a beautiful animal, fur like silk, clear eyed and friendly enough for a house full of children. A year later, when the vet asked Mum if she would adopt Bruno permanently, a very different dog awaited her. In the year between, Bruno had been abandoned and tormented, by children, we presumed, because he feared the young, and was indifferent to the rest. Once a stunning example of his breed, he was now a very sick dog. His fur was eaten away by mange, his eyes were weeping with conjunctivitis, his tail almost hairless. It took every ounce of my mother's healing prowess – turmeric and coconut oil paste applied daily to cure the mange, cotton wool soaked in tea for his eyes, her constant presence by his side – to coax him into a semblance of the show dog he once had been. He did come to enjoy all of us, particularly my father, but his true love would always be my mother.

Certain habits continued to proclaim the fragile state of his psyche. He would habitually walk in circles around our dining table while we ate. Round and round, in an ever-dizzying circumference until, miles clocked up, he would settle somewhere beneath the black glass top.

There was one other place he would circle – the mattress my mother had custom ordered for his bed. At any time of the day or night, he would click clack towards the front door. Slightly to the left of the double doors, he would stop, step onto his fur grubby mattress, turn and turn and turn around, massaging the fabric with his paws, readying his bed for the moment when he would collapse his body, legs first, shoulders second, heavy head upon forepaws last, and then the sigh. Always the sigh. Eyes not entirely closed. His bed faced front and centre. No activity of import could take place without his notice. Even though nothing was required of him, he gave the impression of sleepy vigilance.

My bed, fortunately, does not face the comings and goings of our home life. There is nothing normal about a human taking to their bed at any hour of the day. Sleeping in late into the morning is the reason I was sent to a psychiatrist. Dr. Meyer was worried that I was missing my morning dose of eyedrops due to a combination of insomnia and seeming somnolence; in his concern, he ascribed my lethargy to mental illness. I had no personal stigma against a mental equivalent of physical disease manifesting in me. After all, I had self-diagnosed depression. I just didn't want my mental activity to be placed on weighing scales by figures of authority.

I escaped the psychiatry department, but I never fully freed myself from the guilty association between my relationship to sleep and medical non-compliance, even though my relationship to my bed began not with non-compliance but with the administration of high doses of intravenous and oral steroids. Prednisone would make anyone crazy, if crazy were what you were looking for. Add in daily doses of morphine, and you have Elizabeth Taylor in *Cat on a Hot Tin Roof*, except she's not on the roof, she's house bound, hopping in and around her bed.

To this day, if the hour is late enough, I feel a twinge of something unsettling. Alarm that things are still so far from normal. A quarter to six in the morning and I am still awake. Not widely so. I think I could switch the light off now. The traffic outside is a gentle hum, a soughing wind. The birds have not yet begun. Quick, before the fates decide I am lost, I pack away my wakefulness. And slide down into submission.

There are addictions to my night life. Tidying my Pokémon, for example. Or Candy Crush. I could delete the app. I'm sure I could. But there is something about those brightly coloured candies and the jolly jelly busting fish. And the rewards of a hammer disguised as a lollipop. I play at least five games before bed. After five losses, you have to pay. So, I try to stay within reason. I'm sure there is a connection between the happy candies and my decision to finally let go of the night.

I know I'm not alone in my nightlife. It used to be a more eccentric thing, an artist thing – this staying awake business. But now it's an Everyman who has a smartphone thing. The sky darkens to purple, lightens to mauve, the birds fall silent and then wake, but the world continues to glow and chatter in the palms of our hands. It never stops rewarding us with more and more of whatever we desire and much that we don't. At night is when I go to the school of the globe. I meet my famous friends and I read the encyclopaedia of Wiki wonders. I catch up on the latest articles that Twitter has been kindly accruing for me all day long. And then, since it's morning for them anyway, I message my siblings in Singapore or India to see if anyone's up.

Ever since he could pronounce the word, my nephew Rafael has enjoyed saying he is 'nocturnal' just like his Aunty Shai. At four, he was proud to share this quality with me. At six, his only anxiety was the distance between us. I was living alone at the time. What if I needed him? How would he get from Singapore to Cambridge in time? He especially didn't like the spooky sounds he could hear across the miles. Owls dancing on my roof, I told him. Keeping me company. But maybe they weren't owls. He couldn't see them. He didn't like not knowing. His younger sister, Bella, adopts more of a Guillermo del Toro attitude. Could they be monsters? Let's see!

If it's the twins I get, Ellie or Eva, we discuss mysteries like why Grandma and Papa are in bed sleeping and I am eternally awake. Why is it dark in Cambridge and morning in Bangalore? Would I like a piece of pancake mushed through the phone? Why don't I get on a plane since I'm up anyway and then we can play properly? The circles beneath my eyes deepen into moody maroon bruises and I peel away before 3am. 'Let Shaista sleep now,' says a voice in the background. My siblings are the proper grownups. My position is unclear; variable. 'I'll only go to sleep if there's a grownup in the room,' said Eva to me, negotiating, prevaricating. 'What do you think I am?' I asked. Silence.

But always, always, all four of them will instruct me to wake early.

Once, Eva held my face firmly between her hands, looked seriously into my eyes and said, 'In the morning, when I wake up, wake up early with me, ok? Don't sleep.' And, 'I get tired waiting for you to wake up.' This said without heat or drama. All the more potent for it.

The house is cold now. Radiators temporarily in retirement. I switch my small heater on and contemplate slugging myself to the nearest kettle to boil water for a hot water bottle or a cup of tea. I am hungry. Night-time food is packaged food unless dinner wasn't completely wolfed down. Chocolates and crisps feature now. Occasionally, an experiment. Cheese and tomato ketchup. A fried egg with sesame oil over mixed vegetable rice leftovers. Kimchi, kimchi, where art thou, kimchi?

Sometimes, my first waking thought is this word: death. And just as quickly on its heels: life.

Know this about your chronic illness friends – we are closer to death than you, in thought, but just as busy with life. And because we are alive, we never get used to our closeness to death. Les Murray's poem acknowledges the busyness of bed, how it heralds our screaming arrival, pushes us up and out on bedsprings and legs, and then lays us out, cold, our first grave.

> *You accept my warm absence*
> *There, as you will accept,*
> *One day, my cooling presence…*

Primly dressed, linen-collared one,
You look so still, for your speed,
Shield that carries us to the fight
And bears us from it.

Bed is my yew tree. The place where I heal, the place that heals me. I was born here, and perhaps I will die here, but that doesn't scare me. There is nowhere I would rather be when something, an appointment or social engagement, gets cancelled. The intense relief is a type of nirvana because the lead up to it is arduous. The flip flopping is not as boundless as it once was because my life and the people in it are more streamlined. I know myself more.

But there are still occasions when I force myself forward, thinking it will be alright. I'll manage. I won't fall apart by the side of the road. The ambulance won't have to come for me. So 'I won't die' is often the barometer for going ahead with a plan. But 'I will spend the next several days or weeks surviving the decision' is also part of the barometer.

Calling to cancel a hospital appointment is a tricky business, because NHS appointments are gold dust. And because I've spent so long thinking if I just rest until the last moment, I'll make it. I'm always calculating the mathematical minutes. Working backwards from any appointment. Minutes to get there. Minutes to get a taxi from the point of calling. Possibility for taxi to be stuck in traffic. Minutes necessary for changing out of pyjamas. Minutes spent working out what to wear, what to pack – medicines, reading material for waiting rooms. Food? Have I eaten? When all along my only desire is to be unmoving. A sea urchin upon the bed of the ocean. Coral. You wouldn't know I was breathing unless you lay curled up beside me.

When the phone rings with a social cancelation, there is something specifically personal about the moment – as though the universe really is listening to me with my tiny problems, seeking to find a solution just for me. This is not the truth of it. More than likely someone else is suffering too in that moment – the cancellation, after all, is occurring because someone is ill, or has had bad news. Sometimes you don't know why. But the sweetness of the reprieve is unconcerned with these humanitarian details. *Thank you thank you thank you* is the sleepy sigh that emerges from every intelligent cell. Now we can get back to work – fighting ourselves and fighting inflammation, as always. The business never ends on the inside. On the outside, you may see the twitch of my lips curl into satisfied happiness. The rest of me continues to lie in my bed as though nothing monumental has happened. Only my niece, Ellie, sees through the stillness, into the truth. She draws a picture of me in bed and captions it '*Shaista: Having The Life*'.

You know those dreams where you get up, brush your teeth, eat breakfast, change and walk out? You are on your way and then you wake up to discover yourself still in bed? That, except it isn't a dream. It's my reality. A type of forced sleepwalking, where I wish I were still sleeping. Where bed is the lover I have been forced to leave because reality pulled me away, but my body yearns to return.

LUPUS IN FLIGHT

On the first day of January 2009, I began a blog. I called it 'Lupus in Flight' after a poem I had written as a teenager, soon after my diagnosis.

Lupus in flight,
on a hot and burning night;
would I were the cool breeze,
gliding in and out of sight…

I had been sickening for so long in body and spirit that I was unable to see my way ahead to any sort of future. I became determined to share my poetry. I had by then gathered sixteen journals, one for every year of the disease, and more.

From the first day of the year and on each subsequent day, I posted a poem from the past – the idea being that I would eventually create a chronological body of work, collected in one place, for anyone interested to read the work. After which, death might take me, and I would not look back in regret.

Friends and strangers began to leave comments on my blog. During a four-day February admission, Rizwan lent me his laptop and I began writing new poems to be posted. Late into the night, my fellow inmates fast asleep, I wrote; the knowledge that I had a new life beyond the walls of my hospital room created a vine of hope that I wove tighter around myself with each passing hour. In the months that followed, not knowing how many hours I had left to me, drove out all fear of rejection or self-consciousness. Whenever I could, I dictated letters in the form of blog posts, and either my mother or my brother typed these out for me. And the next morning, or evening, there would be comments awaiting me. Lifelines. The chronology of poetics planned on the first day of the year fell away. Only the raw bones of a life physically confined to hospital remained. The blog saved my life long before the doctors did.

In early March, an ambulance wheeled me back into A&E, and almost immediately onto the Infectious Diseases ward, where every patient has her own room by default, to avoid spreading infection. I had been a shivering mess through the corridors and my mother had wrapped me up in my grandfather's cream Kashmiri shawl. It had been given to me by my grandmother, a precious possession. I must have clutched it to me before the paramedic carried me down the stairs and into the waiting ambulance. Somewhere between transferring my body from the emergency bed to the ward bed, my shawl disappeared. When I discovered its absence, I was bereft. My mother asked the nurses to look for it, but it must have been sent to the laundry for cleaning. I never saw it again.

At first, it looked as though I would slip into a semi-coma, mirroring my entry into the Infectious Diseases ward twelve years earlier. Consultants, registrars, minions loomed around and above me, asking questions, many of which could have been answered by a look at my copious history of notes. I was not on form. Two weeks of fever and dehydration were now clouded by an inexplicable diarrhoea and racking nausea. To counter my dry heaving gags, a nurse injected me with

SHAISTA TAYABALI

'something to help'. A cannula had already been inserted into one of my veins in A&E, so there was no warning or resistance on my part. The 'something to help' turned out to be intravenous Cyclizine, an anti-emetic, which I had always tolerated in tablet form. Intravenous was another matter. I experienced a form of temporary paralysis within minutes. The nurse explained later that she had injected me deliberately to prevent an embarrassing encounter once The Doctors arrived. The anti-emetic was the medical equivalent of a demure, decorous veil being draped over me. God forbid a patient should throw up in the presence of, or worse, on the person of an eminent physician. Instead, I was paralysed. My speech was slurred, my tongue thick, my mind terrified, confused. And the medics watching, noting the patient's inability to speak English clearly. To speak at all. Long after the medics had been and gone, my body relaxed, my ability to move and speak returned and I added IV Cyclizine to my bank of drugs to be avoided: drugs that do not kill you, merely make you wish you were dead.

The fever and diarrhoea marked me out for all sorts of bacterial possibilities, so intravenous antibiotics were prescribed.

On the Infectious Diseases ward, I was subject to a shifting carousel of staff. From my myopic position on a bed in an isolated room, I was never able to gauge the level of experience of the person dealing with me. It was often impossible to know if someone was a health care assistant or a nurse or at which stage of training any of the medics were; even if doctors distinguish themselves between registrar and consultant for you (and they will, because hierarchy is close to godliness in the medical world), you, the patient, don't really understand the stages of years in between. 'Consultant' makes itself the pinnacle by virtue of its rarity, and by the order in which the team presents itself when entering your cubicle or room, and when leaving it. Top brass first, workhorse minnows last. The minnows can become friends. Their interest may begin as academic, research-based thinking (this might make a good

89

paper, someday) but they are the ones most likely to meet your parents, brothers, friends. They may become friends themselves. They may ask to listen to your poetry. And once you've been seen as Poet, you become Shaista again. It gets easier after that.

I like it when my name is known. On March 21st, Parsi New Year, I wrote a poem inspired by one of the housekeeping staff who said, upon hearing my name, 'Shaista. That is a proud name.' He was Lithuanian, and handsome. I enjoyed his visits, his attempts to coax me to eat. After a few weeks, he settled on the one dish I found I was able to tolerate – grated cheese with tiny slivers of pineapple.

I was alive but my body soon became incapable of retaining either fluid or food. I shrank slowly to six stone. And the medical teams began to discuss the necessity of a feeding tube.

There is, for all the obvious financial and time deficit reasons, a lack of attention paid to nutrition in the NHS. Hospitals leave us more mal-nourished than before we enter the corridors. Not many nutrients enter our system while we are in-patients. White bread. Stodgy meat. Potatoes. Ask for fresh salad and it surprises. Fruit is stewed. Rice pudding.

In the beginning, free food cooked by someone else sounds a treat. Regular cups of tea with biscuits seem a godsend. It seems churlish to concern yourself with something so insignificant as meals. The relish with which patients, who can digest their food, look forward to their meals is understandable within the context of not having to cook or think about meals. But the problem manifests itself later in constipation. Elderly patients, trying to pass impossible stools, become the walking dead. Fragile. Pale. No energy to walk. No urgency to walk. Hospitals want and need a quicker turnover. But when we are becoming weaker by the day, what hope is there?

The idea of the feeding tube made me nervous, but I could see there was little point in fighting it. I sat obediently, awaiting the procedure. I did not know that the nurse, who was attempting to manoeuvre the tube up one nostril and down into my oesophagus, had never performed the procedure before. She just wanted to 'have a go'. She was supposed to have a more experienced staff member with her. She was not qualified. I did not know this. When I began vomiting blood, Rizwan could no longer stay silent. He insisted she stop and call a doctor. A doctor was not found, but a woman dressed in a different uniform appeared later in the day. I had to gather my courage for another invasion. I expected more trauma, but the tube went in like silk. Silk, in comparison to the previous three mini-butcherings. Later, my mother reminded me that feeding tubes were nothing new. I'd had them twice before, as a teenager.

I drew the blinds on the window near my bed to discover a concrete block twenty feet opposite my room. The bricks were yellow. Down on the far right, there was a large patch of blue. Was it sky? My eyes couldn't tell. But I pretended it was the sea, reflecting waves at me. I imagined it was the bright blue of Malibu ocean where Jennifer Aniston ran with her dog Norman.

It was Portugal, it was the Maldives.

It was the place of dreams I caught glimpses of in magazines.

Three days after my ode to Jennifer Aniston, the nurse who doled out my medication gave me five times the amount of steroid I normally had. I pleaded with her that I knew how much Prednisone I was supposed to take – I'd been taking the stuff for years. The nurse drew her cape of power tighter around herself, and I became invisible. She insisted she knew better. The doctors knew better – they, after all, had written the prescribed dose. I tried to explain that the doctor, a stranger to my case, must have made a mistake – but clearly this was unheard of in her experience.

My brother took over my blog posts, posting a poem of mine he found lying open on my desk. It was titled 'Snapshots'.

He included this postscript:

Things took a turn for the worse over the past couple of days due to a horrific mistake by the doctors looking after Shaista, and she has not been able to give directions around things to post, so I'm putting this one up for her. Please keep writing in. Every message left here is a happy distraction in a time of a lot of pain and trauma.

Aside from everything else, fevers flare sporadically, various feeds continue, surgical sites haven't stopped hurting yet, and there's a lot of bruising from the myriad punctures of needles; the worst of which appears to be daily warfarin injections straight into the stomach. The pain from these radiates out from point of injection all the way through the body as it works to thin the blood and prevent further clotting. In Shaista's case the bruising then persists, to make the next one even more painful.

Nevertheless, we're seeing snapshots of brightness amidst the gloom and things are looking up a little. Hopefully she'll be back to dictating her own posts very soon. Keep writing in. Thanks, Rizwan.

Between data and flesh, the spirit. Always the spirit. In the midst of physical distress, I recalled that as a nineteen-year old, when death had hovered by my bed, introducing me to my ancestors, I had been given life-saving Intravenous Immunoglobulins as a last resort. Or at least that is how the doctors had presented the drug to me. I was nervous to suggest the treatment now, imagining an instant dismissal. To my surprise, I discovered that funding had, in fact, been procured for me to receive IVIg, but nobody had mentioned this. The golden miracle of immunoglobulin therapy was instated. Twelve bottles of it.

In my next post, I quoted a poem by Thich Nhât Hanh, which begins, '*I hold my face in my two hands/ to keep my loneliness warm... two hands preventing/ my soul from leaving in anger*'. Thây, as he is known to his students, wrote this poem while exiled in France. Bombs were falling on Vietnam, and, helpless as he was, he had to take care of his anger in solitude. I love this poem. It is set to music and sung beautifully by the nuns, especially Sister Chân Không.

My soul was not leaving me in anger, but my body was in trouble even with the addition of IVIg. I was continuing to spike high fevers every night. I spent my days working slowly and mindfully to cool my body. Ice water, paracetamol, breathing, smiling.

One day, I asked my mother to bring some pictures from my bedroom wall at home, of my teachers, my healers, so they could be close beside me. Prophet Zarathushtra, Jesus, Mary, Sai Baba, Thich Nhât Hanh. Although the blinds were drawn for my photophobic eyes, all day long some light would find me. When I asked myself, 'Is this real? Is this really happening?' I would think of my blog, of connections beyond myself and stay purposeful. My room became a magnet for anyone in need of a quiet prayerful moment. Nurses would come in, lean their heads against the image of Mother Mary in her blue cloak, breathe in strength, and walk back, renewed, into their working day. I wondered if management might filter down with warnings against such a display of overt spirituality, but no such warning came.

By Easter Sunday, I had spent forty days on N2, Bay 8. Forty days and forty nights. Wasn't Jesus tested for forty days and nights at Gethsemane? They say prisoners lose their minds after forty days in solitary.

A central line tubing in my jugular was placed successfully but the three access tubes connected to the main catheter weighed heavy on my neck. The days were becoming so unbearable that I too felt I had been abandoned and forsaken by the One I had trusted to watch over me and ease my suffering. Amid high fevers, mouth and throat ulcers, necrotising lymphadenitis, pericardial effusions, thrombophlebitis, and the excruciating tenderness in the wake of a left axilla biopsy, a chaplain visited. The hospital was quiet that Easter, and my room with its clear indication of religious presences, was irresistible. But eventually, her talk of Jesus' suffering on the cross became too much for me, and I had to beg my mother to rescue me from my intense visitor.

I thought back to the self of my first hospital admission twelve years earlier. At eighteen, she thought she was on the brink of something romantic; instead she got needles, toxic drugs, diagnoses of lupus, glaucoma, vasculitis, lymphedema.

I was fighting to pull through, gripping my vine of light. I knew this was the hardest hospital admission of my life, and the most important to get right.

By mid-April, I was able to sit up in the corner chair by the window, straining for the sweet refrain of birds, writing poems of sorrow and joy, despair and hope.

A friend visited and did not like to see the tears in my eyes, my tiredness. 'I am a river of sadness,' I sighed. 'Well, you can't be,' he said, sternly. 'There's no such thing. Rivers move and change and take things away with them and pick things up, like flowers and happiness. Write me a happy poem!'

And eventually, when I had my first walk in too many weeks to count, I did write that happy poem. Arm in arm with my big brother, down to a field of gold I never knew had existed all along, outside the ward. There were bees and butterflies. I wiggled my toes in the cool fresh grass, and unfurled my wings, a little, at last.

By early May, I was writing poems of love, imagining romance a possibility again.

I had had a blood transfusion – two units of lovely, dark, vampirish blood, after which I felt dreamy and peaceful. The feeding tube in my nose had been removed, the catheter from my jugular had been whipped out, and my biopsy site was less painful. The rheumatologists started a new immuno-suppressant called Tacrolimus, because the disease was as yet uncontrolled, sneaky, trying to creep back like ivy, but with none of the old rage and violence. I felt I had the teeth now.

A Rheumatology professor promised me that Tacrolimus was a magic bullet. He was Irish, without any trace of accent (which was suspect), but he said he had written poetry as a boy (which excused him). I wanted to believe in the magic bullet, for him, and not pay any heed to the bloodcurdling list of possible side effects.

'Take no notice of those,' he said. 'It's just obligatory guff.'

To prove how confident he was in the bullet, he sent me home on weekend leave.

Home was all sun and wind, flowers and birds, my parents smiling and relaxed. I slept cosily in my mother's bed, while she slept in my father's bed and he was relocated to the floor of my bedroom.

I thought about nothing in particular. I rested on the garden floor and sang to the colours around me. I kissed petals and avoided the bees. I let the sky examine me, and I ate. My weekly chemotherapy tablet, Methotrexate, had been temporarily stopped to allow the Tacrolimus to work, and suddenly I was in love with food. 'Fish and chips with tartare sauce and tomato slices,' I ordered, bossily. And lo, it arrived (well, my mother made it).

The professor was right, in a way. 129 adverse side effects and the one I developed was not on the list. I began bleeding that weekend. A slow continuous haemorrhage. I knew they would assume it a menstrual discrepancy even though I had recently had my period. But I knew it was a result of the new drug.

Strangely, I felt nothing. No fear, no anxiety. Only my own confidence to match the professor's that I would be proved right and the magic bullet, having proven itself less magical, more violent, would be stopped.

They had promised me monoclonal antibody therapy if Tacrolimus didn't work and that thought alone had me floating. I had such faith in Rituximab and I didn't know why. Nothing had ever worked. No drug had been kind or gentle. And yet, I believed in this drug. The two things can live side by side. Medicine and miracles. The concrete form in pills and surgeries, and the ethereal, the numinous, in that which cannot be spoken, only felt. It doesn't have to be felt alone, it can be shared, but because communication seems invariably to break us down more often than bring us together, miracles are often felt alone. Perhaps the mystical works best, one soul at a time.

Later, back on the ward, something thrilling awaited me. Someone had left a gift in my room while I was home. A mystery! An admirer! My mother, ever practical and damping my ardour, thought it had been forgotten in my room, left behind by mistake, intended for someone else. Thanks, Mum.

I asked all the nurses, and none of them would reveal anything. The gift was a fan, blue and flowered, with sparkly gold stars.

More days passed. I was given a second blood transfusion. I waited to bounce off the walls with strength and energy. But I was too tired to even dictate words of beauty to a silent, sleeping world. I felt strained. Although the Tacrolimus had been stopped, my red blood cells were still haemolysing, breaking up. I had lived on hope for so long, maybe I had worn it thin? A friend sent me a copy of 'The Darkling Thrush' by Thomas Hardy. Reading it reminded me of all I love of life – not least of which is poetry itself and the illimited connections of human beings. Not knowing when we are needed, we suddenly appear. And that moment is the right moment.

The poem was just right. Especially the third verse:

At once a voice arose among
    The bleak twigs overhead
In a full-hearted evensong
    Of joy illimited;
An aged thrush, frail, gaunt, and small,
    In blast-beruffled plume,
Had chosen thus to fling his soul
    Upon the growing gloom.

To fling my soul upon the growing gloom is all I ever want to do.

My Lithuanian friend on the housekeeping staff turned out to be the mysterious fan giver. He had been to Venice with his girlfriend over the long bank holiday weekend and chosen something sparkling with the promise of holidays for me. I received the gift in the spirit it was meant, but some of the younger female staff decided to tease me. One of them told me, 'You can have a boyfriend, if you want one.' I gave her an odd look. 'Do you know how old I am?' I asked. She double checked my wristband. Shock. Then discomfort. She was at least eleven years younger than me.

I was thirty years old when I decided I'd had enough of being patronised.

By the end of May, they had paved the green beyond my blinds. The blue gorse and heather I had mistaken for sky or ocean were gone. It was time to leave the four walls of my room behind. I was discharged just before June arrived, eighty-four days after being admitted.

Over the summer, I was given my first rounds of Rituximab, the new chemotherapy I had been promised for months. At first, it raged a storm in me, violent rashes spread over my skin in raised rivers of itching. The itching left me breathless, the hunger to itch equally so. It can be a fascination – the way a drug casts a curse over your flesh. Bewitching. The slow quick rise of fever. Your lungs constricting, your flesh changing colour, texture. I spent the weeks in between rounds, at home, burning, burning.

In the autumn, I wrote a poem called 'The Year of Yes'. The only reason I was able to write a poem of *Yes* is because I had finally learnt to say *No*. To incompetence, to the power hungry, to those who were happy to gamble with my life. Something had awakened in me. In those eighty-four days, I learned that I loved my life. I loved this Shaista girl who had become a woman. Learning to say *No* that year was my Patronus charm: how to save your life by coming to your own rescue.

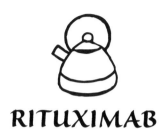

RITUXIMAB

I n 2011, two years after I began receiving Rituximab, America began the process of approving the first treatment that might possibly offer a solution to the incurable nature of lupus.

It is called Benlysta or Belimumab (who thinks up these names?) and it is an investigational human monoclonal antibody therapy drug. Mabtherapy. Since Rituximab is also monoclonal antibody therapy, I must be on the right track. I know I am. *So* close.

But it is such a fight to 'deserve' the treatment. And be a good investment for the high risk.

You find yourself fighting for a possible future you don't know exists, trying to prove the worth of your individual soul to a near stranger, a figure of authority, within fifteen minutes, without descending into emotion, becoming antagonistic, or losing hope.

Heart, soul and poetry have little place in the consulting rooms of a Head of Department in charge of funding. A medical degree would be brilliant, but even that is no guarantee. What does that leave? A sense of dread? A sense of humour?

What you need is exceptionality.

Here is a definition of medical exceptionality:

In order to demonstrate exceptionality the patient must be significantly different from the reference population (i.e. all other patients with the same condition who do not fulfill the treatment criteria) and there must be good grounds to believe that this patient is likely to gain significantly more benefit from this intervention than might be expected for the average patient with that condition. The fact that the treatment might be efficacious for the patient is not, in itself, grounds for exceptionality. This in essence requires the clinician to make a case why this particular patient should be funded when others will not receive treatment.

– from the First National Immunoglobulin Database Report (2008-2009)

It is easier to confer exceptionality on others, harder to prove one's own. What is my worth in funding? One morning, after I had the all-important funding-dependent blood test to check the depletion levels of my B-cell lymphocytes, I asked the consultant why this test was not done regularly on me. She said it cost £100. I did not know how to respond. I never know how to respond when given concrete sums against which I have to determine my worth.

In my mind I keep hearing this song: *How much is that doggy in the window? The one with the waggly tail?* That is what it has come down to for me. *How much is that Shaista in the window? I do hope there's more to her tale.*

The painful irony of fighting to qualify for Rituximab or Belimumab is the reel of side effects. On the Benlysta website, under important healthcare information, is a trilogy of statements resembling a Japanese koan:

Benlysta can cause serious side effects.
Some of these side effects may cause death.
It is not known if Benlysta causes these serious side effects.

The list of reasons to not take such a drug is almost unnecessary when faced with the simplest side effect of death. Here, try this drug. It might kill you, or it might not. No human who wants to live should ever have to be given a drug that might cause death, but that would rule out almost every single drug prescribed for lupus.

It certainly rules out Rituximab. Before being given my first infusion of the drug, I googled it. And read the case history of the patient who died from PML (progressive multifocal leukoencephalopathy), the brain infection you become more susceptible to on cytotoxic immune weakening therapy. And yet, I trusted in the drug. The slightly magical, loving relationship I have with Rituximab continues, eleven years later. Nothing untoward, beyond manageable infections, has turned up so far, but we keep checking.

The drug is given in two rounds, two weeks apart. The first round is always worse. The first day after is an uphill strain, a run after months of slovenly unfitness. Your heart sulks but works hard to pump life and toxicity, with alternate beats.

The second day, the fevers nestle in. The heating is on, your electric blanket switches on and off, but the cold and the heat of the chemo flush, dance to a tune all their own.

The third day, less of the fevers. Now it's the breathing you struggle with. A chubby hedgehog is sitting between your lungs, stretching yogi bear poses into your ribs. You gasp, open mouthed, catching air.

You boil water for tea, coffee, hot water with lemon. You try to keep hydrated at least, so you don't have to process food into a system already overworked.

Backache, hunched over a keyboard. Straining eyes against fading winter light. The kettle pings, and you drag yourself over. You think of Zen Buddhist monks and nuns, you picture a little temple surrounded by koi fish in a pond, and ancient tortoises, or are they turtles? Tea ceremonies. A holy ritual for all of us, even if later, once the pouring is done, the scent inhaled, your steam caressed nose and cheeks cool, you throw away three quarters of undrunk liquid, tasteless now.

You fight the light. In your mind, you hustle your entertainments together, sifting quickly through your choices. A movie? A magazine? An episodic comedy or drama from Netflix? They all require your eyes. Your left optic nerve winces at the pressure you intend to inflict upon it. Audiobook? Radio? You could close your eyes.

You close your eyes. And darkness descends. Too soon, you think. It will be dark soon enough and closing your eyes only hurries the inevitable.

Your thumping heart pounds at the door of your chest. You listen for a while. And even though it's only late afternoon, there is a chorus of anxious birdsong on the other side of your skylights. The fog is settling in.

Eventually, you succumb. You put your contact lenses in. Everything comes into sharp focus. You notice how many things you have. It shocks you. What are you going to do with all these things if you die suddenly? How will all these things be disposed of?

You force yourself to commit to something, anything, however trivial, so the enormity of your mortality does not overwhelm you. You have been here before, many times, and it is because you are still here that you have acquired these things. They are beautiful, each in their own way, each telling a story of how they came to be. Many of them are gifts. Handmade bags from Mexico, India and Zambia. A portrait drawn by your brother. A lifetime of books, bought and loved. Although the messy spills across every flat surface embarrass you, the freedom with which these things co-habit, inspires you. And finally, you sleep.

Day 4 post chemo and I feel I have woken too early. I wait for what feels like hours before checking my phone for the time. A quarter past eight. The whole day lies ahead of me. I climb through the hours in stages of bed, tea, a piece of fruit, chocolate and Benedict Cumberbatch in 'Parade's End'. I am straining my eye muscles, my optic nerves, but the alternative is too heavy today. The fever is higher today. I am horribly cold and force myself to the bathroom only when the pressure on my bladder becomes too great. I think about romance and marriage, as I always do when I am at my most crumpled, and any future beyond a lifetime in bed seems impossible. I try to remind myself of Elizabeth Barrett, but although I can picture her stretched out on her chaise longue, being emotionally traumatised by her father, I cannot picture Robert Browning in a heroic light. And not because Emma Thompson and Stephen Fry's spoof has left its mark of mockery. I have never been able to see him clearly.

I, like many others before me, immediately identified with Jo in *Little Women*, but Beth is the one I have most resembled. We wonder about Beth's inner life; what lives alongside the saintliness? Even Jo is fooled. Even Jo believes Beth is secretly enamoured of Laurie, yearning for an impossible love. Beth was never fooled. She knew she was dying, and so did her mother, who made plans for all her daughters, except Beth.

That is the kernel of a life like mine. I exist somewhere between Beth and Elizabeth. I am Shaistabeth. A Beth of both. Not quite dying, nor being swept into a wild romance with a fellow poet.

Louisa May Alcott, the Philadelphian abolitionist, feminist and novelist, is thought to have had lupus, though it was never diagnosed. Unlike Jo, who surprises herself with a husband and children, Alcott never married.

We, the ill, do marry, or are already married. We fall in love, we make love. And babies. Wriggling, living, demanding. But on day 4 of a Rituximab cycle, my body is fit for no one else. I am in constant awe, and no little anxiety for the mothers I meet on the ward; their children visit with a vivid energy that is shushed almost instantly. I try not to project what I might have felt had I been three or nine years old, and my mother were stretched on a narrow white bed with a tube snaking into her flesh.

Once, I watched a mother and daughter on the ward. When her mother was free of the IV and standing up, the daughter, who was much taller, tenderly tidied her mother's hair, straightened her jacket, tucked her into a wheelchair. The mother said something to her daughter in Urdu. I wanted to ask her to speak louder, so I could hear her words of love. But I didn't. I pretended to be invisible.

I find I cannot quite meet the eyes of the husbands, boyfriends, partners in the monotony of hospital life. I am afraid I will see boredom, fear, disgust, frustration. But the fact of their physical presence ought to make me trust. Love makes itself felt by being present, does it not? Its presence energises the room or sobers it. While she sleeps, he reads a book, but her needled hand is held warm in the clasp of his free hand.

The only way I can envisage romantic love is as a conversation begun and continued. An endless meandering conversation. This, I think I can handle.

Day 5. Roiling nausea. Paracetamol rarely has the power to control lupus fevers. A GP once explained to me the logic of taking four pairs of paracetamol tablets every day to control fever. It builds up a level in your blood, he said, that will prevent the fever from spiking. I always try advice. I can't remember how many pairs I survived before vomiting them up. The GP never mentioned they might add to my already fractious state of nausea.

I make myself a cup of tea. I am drowning in tea. I keep food down with determination to soothe my mother's plaintive, 'Have you eaten?'

Must I eat? Is it so important?

I close my eyes and step inside an imaginary cubicle. Light floods through me. Liquid gold.

But it's no good. Dramatic measures are called for. I need a real cubicle, not a visualised one. I need actual liquid. It takes a certain measure of courage to face the undressing, and then the dreaded seconds post heat, into towels, and finally socks, and other warming, bundling things. Inside of a shower, I can pretend I am as normal as anyone, concentrating only on scrubbing my scalp, scenting vanilla, imagining I am preparing for an evening out. I am careful, keeping in mind how dangerous bathroom accidents are, but it never fails. Even in hospital, especially in hospital, the regeneration of hot water and soap is miraculous.

Freshly showered, I turn the corner. I see moments from the future. I make a small plan. But still, my body hurts. My right supraclavicular lymph node swells and deflates, fever rises and falls. And in a week, I will present myself to the chemo dragon juice once more.

On my return, another dance begins. 'Now,' my mother says, hands not necessarily on hips, but sounding as though they are: 'What do you want to eat?'

Food is the battleground of our love.

Food, we are told, in every documentary and from every well-meaning relative across the pond, is the answer, is the cure. Make her juices. Give her more flaxseeds. Coconut oil. Apple cider vinegar.

But when your daughter is cowering in bed with the shakes and her bruised eyes are begging you not to force her into collaborations over meal plans, your head goes a little fuzzy. By evening, it is my mother who has retired to her bed, and curled up, hoping like a child that when she wakes, the curse some rogue witch left upon her precious daughter will have been lifted and the face greeting her above the sheets will be sparkly and smiling.

Only it isn't. What greets her is the oldest face of despair. The sparkle has gone. Was it ever there long enough? Your mother cannot remember when the sparkle last visited. She has her own anxieties. Her own health concerns. Her CT scan to check for a possible cancer is due the day after.

I, in my toxic state, am determined to keep her company, but I know, in the morning, she will whisk herself off before I have a chance to do more than wave a feeble arresting hand, and croak, 'I'm coming. I just need a few... more... minutes...'

The face of despair has been reincarnated here in this house in Bletchley Park type permutations. But so has it also been overcome. So finely tuned are we three to the nature of despair, that the subtle trill of humour or the deft interweaving of a little light, is transformative. Transient transformations are what we live for here.

Meanwhile... death, death, death, I think in a steadying march. Where else but death could any of this lead? It is 4:38am and dawn seems to be whistling herself into readiness for day. You don't want to catch the transition. It'll be unbearable, so perky. You force yourself to switch the lamplight off just before the birds come calling, and with any luck, the next hell that awaits you must be woken into. But that's hours and miles of sleep away.

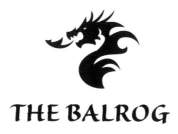

THE BALROG

You don't know it's coming for you. You don't see it coming. For years, you travel in directions signposted by blood work reports, body temperature and levels of infection. One year slides meekly in behind another year in your file, and somewhere along the way you pause and think, this could be it. If this is as good as it gets, you'll take it.

You don't mean it. You want it to be better, but you're trying a new tactic of not imagining the worst. You deal with the low-lying anxieties. You believe they are natural consequences of a near lifetime of physical illness and the particular shade of vulnerability that comes with myopia and glaucoma.

And then, one day, an ulcer is born on the surface of your eye.

I had just turned twenty-seven. Keith had been unable to resuscitate my left eye trabeculectomy and my eye was still healing from the Molteno implant operation he had finally had to perform. I remember the hours of relentless optic nerve torture that had led up to the operation. But with the corneal ulcer, I wanted to die, over and over again. Suicidal ideation, I think it's called. But I'm not sure it gets me anywhere knowing the term.

I want to die as much as I want to live. I don't want to live in quite this way, and I don't want to die any old way. We all think about dying in the midst of living but mental and physical wellness tip the scales in favour of living. It's so delightful to be alive and eating or walking or reading or even arguing for the sake of watching language form itself on your tongue in neat, clever arrangements.

The balance of life and death is disrupted by chronic illness. The constant hum of fear and anxiety running beneath the surface of your flesh, conversing inside of veins and in pockets of auto-antibody molecules, roars out of you soundlessly one day, waking you up to the possibility that you were wrong, you don't actually want to live at all. There were reasons, but they are all feeble. Look at them, shrinking and losing all texture even as you command them to hold still and speak up for themselves.

At the heart of depression lies its most negative seed: the memory of what we were once capable of doing, of enjoying, compared with the loss of it now. This seed multiplies feelings of despair into an endless graph of exponential future defeats. It is difficult enough coping with what has come to be, but we are experts at pushing the boat further into what will come to be, by a simple, abusive act of imagination. Not *this might get worse*, but *this will surely get worse*. In the land of predictive text of our brain, we never seem to be able to write wonder and optimism. The optimist is considered a naïve fool. The pessimist is a realist until he tips himself over into depression, then he must once again correct, over correct by pursuing happiness. We rarely get the balance right.

Upon diagnosis, the sick person becomes boatman to the boat owned by death. We do not want to be on this boat. We want to ascribe to a different worldview, without illness, pain, gunshot wounds, shrapnel. The myth of the sick person salutes the brave patient, assuming a point of courage has been reached and maintained, but we, the sick, find no comfort in this. We know how easily we can be reduced to less than human. Case notes. Numbered levels of pain and data.

The sick person is a seer in some ways. She knows illness is coming for you, healthy ones. It is a kind of psychic torture we live with. We, who live inside this skin, cannot, even with our mythical insights and knowledge, protect or prevent disease in others. It may be called by another name – Alzheimer's, Parkinson's, cancer, stroke – or simply the nature of ageing, for which none of us are prepared; when the healthy are healthy, they cannot understand the life of the sick, and when the healthy are no longer their healthy selves, they may have little time for the sick. The chronically sick person is lonely, always.

The sick person dreads war and old age. Looming burdens, neither of which may occur. Dying young is not ideal, but a tethered life – always dependent on medicines, on help – is its own prison.

Imagining romance becomes difficult at this point. Knowing illness is coming, one hopes to at least have had a happy foundation of escapades unleavened by disease. Someday, joints curled by arthritis, left arm paralysed by stroke, one would prefer to look back over a life well lived and taste the sweet beside the bitter. But perhaps we are all on the outside, looking in, to other lives, which appear greener and merrier than our own?

My mother has a saying: *cross that bridge when you come to it.* But inherent in the saying is the sting of *when*. That bridge will come. If not that bridge, then another. But the bridges will come. Fear is twinned with lupus. They thrive together, feeding succulently on each other. People speak of the power of the mind, but no one mentions the part about how long it takes to disempower fear and engage directly with the wolf. Meanwhile we play the butterfly, the social dance we perform in company and sometimes, more often than we care to admit, to ourselves.

They say calling a thing by its name is an act of power, of ownership. I have not found this to be true in the case of depression. 'Depression' does not encompass the experience of the thing itself. It is merely the portal to the beast within. Hence the necessity of metaphorical language, like 'the black dog'. But 'the black dog' would not be my choice to describe the beast.

When I was a child reading Enid Blyton and Roald Dahl, Tolkien's trilogy never came my way. Depression was deeply embedded in my daily battle with glaucoma when the first of the Peter Jackson films, *The Fellowship of the Ring*, was released in cinemas. But it was not until after my corneal ulcer took residence on the surface of my left eye, and I turned to the audiobook recordings of *The Lord of the Rings*, that I drew specific meaning from the battle between Gandalf the Grey, and the Balrog.

Gandalf, the mighty wizard, is dragged into a deep chasm by the flame of Udûn, burned, frozen and devoured by the Shadow, until, upon his victory, he emerges, healed, clothed in white, as Gandalf the White, more powerful than before. I don't believe the last part is particularly true for us non-wizards, but the seemingly endless battle in the chasm with an unseen shadow is true enough. You never emerge the same. Something has been taken from you. And you will always live in fear of those vast, shadowy wings. All you can do is stay vigilant to the signposts and find ways to distract, amuse and quiet the tremulous part of you that remembers.

I run baths.

I run baths because they take time. The whole endeavour can last up to an hour or more. I have to talk myself out from under the duvet where fever has sweated out of me in rivulets of toxicity. The pressure I place on the bath is intense. I need it, not simply to cleanse my body of superficial toxins and dead cells, I need it to cure death, disease and depression.

The water needs to be scalding. I remember bathing from a bucket in Mahableshwar, the hill station where we vacationed as children. It was so cold in the bathroom, that water seemed to lose heat the instant it left the cosy confines of the bucket to touch our naked, whimpering skin. *Quick! Quick!* Sweaters awaited us, warm corduroy trousers, bed under a mosquito blanket. And books.

I inch my way in. No pity for my flesh which may be red and raw afterwards but that's the least of its worries. The left side of my body from eye to foot is tight. It has had more trauma than the right. My right leg can do nothing but efface itself. I find this unhelpful and force myself to say, *how lovely and relaxed you are, right leg.* I am trying to encourage the two disparate sides of my body to communicate. But the left will have nothing to do with softness.

I slide down and become a frog, legs bowed out, feet angled in. I let the water lap at me between my legs, a moving, kissing thing. I wait, hopeful that the anxieties of my left side will melt over to the right, and the joyful freedom of the right will fool the left. It does for a few seconds. I am safe here, door locked from the outside world.

But the outside world filters in. Dad bellows, 'Hello? Everything alright?' I don't think he's really worried, although I have been in here a while, so I don't blame him. I call out, 'Yes!' or 'Fine!' How normal my voice sounds. So alive! Where does it come from, this lovely, normal sound? It amazes me every time I speak that I can speak.

'*Hello?*' he calls, again. He isn't checking I'm alive. He's check- ing he's alive. 'Hello' has long been my father's code word for asking: 'Everything alright?' 'How about a cup of tea?' 'Anything funny to listen to? I'm a bit desperate right now.'

We have an evening date to attend to, my father and I. Between 5:30 and 6pm we crawl out of our dens and meet in the kitchen by the kettle. I boil water, make tea, arrange biscuits, and we converse in brief, broken sentences. Sometimes I read the latest Mma Ramotswe aloud, while Dad drinks tea and eats Ritz crackers with cheese. Sometimes we fight, like the time he insulted me saying he and I could never write a book (no patience, unlike Mum) and to my self-piteous, 'What's the point?' he countered, 'Frida would never say that – she would fight on, wheeled out in her bed!'

Frida Kahlo was eighteen when a near fatal bus accident crushed her, breaking her spine, collarbone, ribs, shoulder, piercing her abdomen. For almost thirty years, she painted her beautiful and bloody reality. Then, a year before her death in 1954, gangrene set in, and doctors amputated her right leg below the knee. In her diary, Frida drew her feet and wrote,

> '*Pies, para que los quiero, si tenga alas pa' volar?*'
> '*Feet, what do I need you for, when I have wings to fly?*'

I find myself wondering whether Kahlo would have written the same sentiment if her eyes, rather than her feet, had been called into question. *Eyes, what do I need you for, when I have…?* She would have. She was brave enough for that.

By six, I am somewhat patched together by sugar and Dad's comforting or invigorating presence, and I retire to sit in front of the television for twenty minutes of *Strictly Come Dancing: It Takes Two*. Zoe and the glitter ball carry me forward just enough to believe I am here in the same life as these smiling, dancing humans. Maybe it will be alright.

But first, I must leave the sanctuary of this bathroom with its scalding time-out. Another end to pretending I am three years old when bath time promised the beginning of playtime or bedtime.

A key turns in the lock downstairs. My mother is home. My father perks up like our golden retriever Bruno used to when an apple was peeled. Or a banana. Although bananas often signalled sneakily concealed tablets, so he was slightly cautious in his excitement.

There is no caution in the way my father yells out my mother's name.

She calls out my name first. There is no asking how I am, even though a question mark rests after my name; she knows how I am. She has been out and done the things that need to be done to keep the house ticking along. Somewhere in her parcels, there will be a little something for me. A magazine. A slice of cake. A whole cake, depending on how haunted my eyes had looked before she left the house.

The kettle sings and a tray arrives. My parents enter into the conversation that has been ongoing since they met. It doesn't have any beginnings or endings. It just goes quiet now and then, when they fall asleep, or someone leaves a room, or my mother switches the TV on to unwind.

Meanwhile, I face the rising. The temperature above the water level must be confronted. I am aware of leaving an old skin behind in the tub. I slither out of it. I have escaped something, again.

When I emerge, they are discussing people I don't know, and then people I do know, from a book. As my father crunches into a pistachio cookie, he remembers a line. 'How comfortable it is to have macaroons for tea!' He is quoting *A Civil Contract* by Georgette Heyer. Famous for her Regency romances, this novel is, for Heyer, a uniquely real look at a marriage that begins with unrequited love but ends in true harmony. Adam, Sixth Viscount of Lynton, thinks it a coincidence that he arrives home in time for fresh macaroons, unaware that Jenny keeps the cook on tenterhooks awaiting her lord's arrival, and the macaroons have been freshly baked every day in case his lordship should take the fancy.

Is it intentional or unintentional, this innocent discussion? I am grateful, whichever it is.

Sometimes I walk down the corridor past my father's study and hear laughter, music. I open the door to find my parents half-waltzing, half-swinging around the tiny room. 'It's Magic Mix on the radio!' my father shouts over the music, and I watch with a cheesy smile, as I have always done since memory began – my parents talking in a dance, just walking in a dance, through this thing called marriage.

WARDS AND WARDENS

When I watched *The Shawshank Redemption,* I recognized a familiar kernel of truth.

Even when released from prison, Morgan Freeman's character Red needs to ask permission from his new employer before he can go to the bathroom and relieve himself. I know what it is to be used to asking whether I need to hand in a sample: of fluid, of flesh. Different reason. Similar lasting psychological effect.

Hospitals are not, in their natural state, a place of friendliness. Or charm. Women growl in here, their deep lowing unrecognisable as human voices. Smiles are suspect. If you're smiling, you're not really ill. You don't really know pain. A smile suggests you are a fraud.

There are clocks everywhere, white circles of timekeeping in a place run by time, where people are destroyed by time. The hours commit you. Sanity and insanity beat alternative counts, keeping rhythm with churning infusion pumps and a cacophany of snores. Inside of time, women snore safely, falling away into secret places. There is always a voice calling, 'Help! Help!' It paces itself in the repetition of the word, drawing out the 'he-ell', the soft plosive 'p' seems only added for effect, until the word becomes whole, becomes a howl. In your mind, you picture the body-in-torment, on the floor perhaps, scrabbling for the sides of their bed, and you are close, only in the next room and yet you are too far, from a body-mind so ravaged it cannot help itself. You should be compassionate and rush to pick the body up, but you don't. You are attached to tubes. You hold your breath and listen, waiting for the end of the howl, for help to come. Sometimes, you press your buzzer and under pretext of asking for some minor thing, quietly point out that there is a person in torment somewhere close by, and had they, the nursing staff, heard?

Sometimes, the howl is wordless. And vaguely or actually threatening. 'If you don't come to me NOW, hell will break loose her furies. And you will be damned.' No one comes. No one fears damnation here. We, patients and nursing staff, are already in varying levels of hell.

Women fall. The ambulance comes. Clothes are removed from bodies and replaced by faded scraps someone decided to call 'gowns' – a cruel joke, for what resemblance do these shapeless, dignity erasing items bear to the long, floating dresses worn by wealthy women of earlier generations? Dentures may be forgotten in the rush. Hairbrushes are never packed, or lipstick, or shoes. Spectacles, books, knitting, address books with friends and relatives' numbers. All the pieces that mark our unique selves, that separately connect us. I lie beside the dentureless, the hopelessly bored, the blurry-eyed, lipstickless; unadorned, we are less women, more data than flesh. We are first names – Dorothy – without surnames, without lineage. Our birth dates are useless here, except to provide ammunition for those who wish to patronise us. And we discover this: a woman can be patronised at any age.

We are moved, pawns on a chess board, from test to test. Tests we have not arranged. The day unfolds according to plans made without either our approval or knowledge. A wheelchair suddenly arrives to take us from the ward, from the bed that has become home, into the outside world of the corridors, the long cold roads that shock us into awareness of our sick selves. We pass the walking, the visiting, the dressed-normally.

We can gauge the weather outside from the dressed-normally. We smell coffee and burgers, floating scents. We salivate for our old lives.

A woman died behind my head one night. She had been a thumper for days and nights, battering vengeance into our shared wall. Irfan had made jokes about her to assuage his own fears, as well as my anxieties. He didn't like leaving me alone with the crazy thumping lady, feet away from me. A wall divided us, but doors remain unlocked on the wards. At night, before he left, we laughed about her together, my brother and I. The next day, when all was quiet, I thought she had heard us. I felt wracked with guilt and grateful all at once. But by evening, when Irfan visited again, I had news. She wasn't offended. Or attending to my needs. She was dead.

Minds lose themselves in here. My brother's fears were based on known specific tales. One night, I had woken to find the elderly lady from the bed diagonally opposite mine, clawing at my bed sheets and cawing at nothing in particular. Her gown was lifted. She was poised and ready, to urinate or defecate, I'll never know which, because a nurse arrived in time to muscle her away from my bed to the real toilet. Later, the nurse came to find me and apologise, but no explanation was ever given for what I simply learned to accept: *some patients have dementia.* And those four words must suffice.

I had just turned nineteen the first time I was admitted onto a women's ward under the aegis of Rheumatology. The majority of patients were elderly, arthritic, and dementia seemed an almost casual accident of the experienced long-term hospital inmate.

Dementia doesn't justify racism, but when the same patients were racist and wandering loose, I had to learn early on not to take offence or lose my footing when instructions were barked at me. Walking from bed to bathroom and back again, I was invariably asked in varying tones of irritation or cajoling, to fill water jugs, clean bed pans, and why was I not wearing my uniform? Because my skin colour seemed to indicate I must be either domestic or nursing staff.

One week after America's World Trade Centre was bombed, I was admitted to hospital. On the ward with me, was a woman named Mary. It hurt to watch her move, breathe; her pain felt so tangible. She was over eighty, and rheumatoid arthritis was crippling her. From time to time, I fetched her water when I could see she needed it. She often mistook me for a nurse, in spite of the fact that I occupied the bed opposite her.

One day, my friend Leo visited with Rizwan. Leo's face was almost obscured by the birds of paradise in his arms. I had been in need of beauty.

We began receiving the strangest looks from across the room. Leo is over six feet and Haitian, my brother a tall Indian. We, all three of us, received the strangest looks.

After the two of them left, the tension was palpable on the ward.

Later, Mary had visitors – they brought the day's papers filled with images of suspected terrorists – and her voice carried, devastating me. I had never had such vitriol directed at me. Or such fear. She was scared of me. The irony was this: I knew her name but she didn't know mine; the way my name carries my heritage should have been doubly alarming to her. Names mean everything in India. Names give away your hiding place, reveal your religious identity to men ready to burn down your home. But names are unnecessary information in England, when your face, your skin, is enough of a calling card.

I tried to spend time outside the ward, in the reading room. But I was ill too and exhausted with carrying the weight of her burden of fear. She wanted me to go back to where I came from and take the evil and wickedness with me.

I wanted to go home too. Where was that?

A person of colour does not enter the world thinking of herself as a person of colour. I was at university when I finally found the language to express race awareness. My bachelor's degree in English Literature at Cambridge's Anglia Ruskin University was modular, so for the first time I was able to choose my education, tailor it to my interest. It was a thrill discovering Alice Walker, Ntozake Shange, Maya Angelou, Toni Morrison (almost all the writers I was drawn to self-identified as women of colour), and I began to see that the colour of my skin preceded me, an identity card I had no control over. It also made me feel more isolated because with knowledge came insight. I had lived through the first years in England forcing myself to believe my mother when she promised me the bus drivers and shop girls were not moved by prejudice or racism, but instead were having 'bad days'.

Seeing myself as immigrant has been a complicated process of sifting past negative associations and finding beauty in our individual and collective narratives. In England, immigrant is a word loaded with negative connotations – powerful ones to do with theft of property, of the national soul. You immigrant, you have come here to take away from us. So, go back, go far away, back to your land. Our land is not your land.

A childhood memory comes to me of singing these lyrics with my Californian cousin Emily, belting them out with gusto: '*This land is your land, this land is my land, from California to the New York island*' and not knowing then what Thanksgiving really meant, believing the spirit of the song, believing in the America of that song.

To me, the word 'immigrant' means story. I credit Chitra Banerjee

Divakaruni and Amy Tan with teaching me this. The immigrant is an unfinished novel in human form. The child of immigrant parents, carries this novel with her and feels compelled to give the novel an ending fit for kings and queens – wealth, property, success – but when, instead, she finds herself seeking happiness, the novel becomes more complicated than ever. In pursuit of personal happiness, the immigrant story becomes an ordinary story once more – the story of any man, any woman, trying to be human. It is revolutionary in most of the old cultures to be an artist or sportswoman not because the culture does not support these professions, but because arts and sport offer the chance for visibility, for the old stories to be told in our mouths, on our tongues, and not by the appropriation of others.

I took a life drawing class during my first year at university. I drew a woman whose skin was pierced and tattooed. Her body introduced me to my first experience of tattoo as art in England. Tattoos in India, as with tribal cultures, have meanings, claimed identities. I began to see something of this cultural continuation here in my new land. My lecturer, Simon Featherstone, introduced excerpts from the 1994 New Zealand film *Once Were Warriors* as part of his tutorial. It remains one of the most powerful films I have ever seen. At the time, I became deeply absorbed by a series of mythological Maori female narratives. I drew breasts in hillocks, bellies as mountaintops, bottoms curving deep into the core of the earth. I saw the connections between Indian goddesses, like the goddess of war, Durga Mata, and Latina archetypes of Mother Earth, in the works of Sandra Cisneros, controlling mud, winds, the dark.

Alongside 'immigrant', I discovered 'Asian': an umbrella term for people who come from my part of the world. I found it an equivalent laziness to describing someone as African. Accurate and inaccurate in equal measure. At Peter Taylor, my university hall of residence, a group of British Asians tried to draw me into their fold. I was grateful but could not share their rhythm. I felt just as much of an outsider with them because I am not the second-generation child of first-generation immigrants. I am the migrant. I found the terms 'British' and 'Asian' alone, or together, a new uncomfortable skin. I could not join in the mockery, however affectionate, of Indian accents, Indian ways. It was too close to the bone. I was missing home. I was missing home.

By the final year of my BA, I knew exactly what I wanted to explore for my dissertation. I had come to believe that racial and sexual violence creates a need in women for freedom, which can only be found in the spiritual self. I decided to focus on the American South, traveling from Zora Neale Hurston to Flannery O'Connor and meeting them both in Alice Walker.

Walker's definitions of 'womanism' – '*usually referring to outrageous, audacious, courageous or wilful behaviour*' and '*wanting to know more and in greater depth than is considered 'good' for one*' – initiated me into the feminist movement by way of the narratives of women of colour. And yet, immersed as I was in raced and gendered reading, in the days following my graduation, I had to make a choice to either divorce or embrace the whiteness in me. I realized my feminism was a womanist feminism. A black brown white feminism. Every character in my early stories, as a child writer in India, had been white without whiteness being a thing I was aware of – they were named Primrose and Jane because those were the names of heroines in the books I read. I didn't think Primrose and Jane were better human beings than me. I didn't think Primrose and Jane could be heroines but Shaista could not. Shaista was the ultimate heroine since she had her name on the cover of the book. She was the creator of the book.

I have been the only brown skinned girl in the same English village for over twenty years. Inside my own bubble, I am everything. Articulate, intelligent and committed to equality. Outside the bubble, my tongue gets twisted into knots by social circumstance. *Do you feel this is your home now? Or is India still your home?* Home is where you are never asked this question. But I am too polite to say this out loud. Politeness creates barriers of silence. In England, I am ever conscious of following the unbreakable code of guest in a host country, the complete opposite of what you might experience on coming to India where you, *mehman* (guest), are also *Bhagwan* (God).

For myself, I want only to be the most authentic brown girl dreaming. To know and love the taste, the scent, of my own bones and shadows. And be unapologetic about inhabiting my skin. Race relations demand apologies on both sides. *Why are you the way you are? Can't you be more like me?* In my experience, sharing race-based anecdotes turns reality into stories. Stories offer possibilities of believing or disbelieving in characters, choosing loyalties, questioning veracity, objectivity.

I have shared anecdotes of racism only a handful of times with English friends, and every time I have watched my friend slip away, pulled away by stronger ancestral bloodlines. The question of race makes us tribal. Modern manners fall away and something older, fiercer, takes hold of us. The once powerful remember their pride. The newly powerful dig their heels in, grinding The Others to dirt beneath their feet.

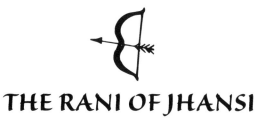

THE RANI OF JHANSI

In the comments section of my blog, I am often referred to as Warrior Poet.

In one of my poems, I claim it myself:

I am standing on the battleground, listing a little,
sword and pen at the ready, blood and words aplenty…

The idea of being a warrior was first planted when I saw an image of Rani Lakshmi Bai of Jhansi in a history textbook at school, instantly recognising bravery in the illustration of the nineteenth century queen, sword in hand, astride a horse. Did I know for sure why she impressed me and none of the illustrious men in my history books did? Was it the singularity of the image or a deeper understanding of who she was, how she came to be? She was a freedom fighter against the injustices of the British, tying her son to her back, reins in her mouth, a sword in each hand, plunging into a battle to the death.

The Rani of Jhansi is not the only historically famous Indian female warrior – Rani Abbakka Chowta, a sixteenth century warrior queen from a matrilineal lineage, was the only woman to confront and repeatedly defeat the Portuguese – but the presence of just one woman in warrior garb was enough to make a lasting impression on me, so that years later when I found myself hailed as warrior poet, I didn't think it an oxymoron or a metaphorical fiction. Women have been warriors throughout history, across the globe. We just don't see it represented enough. But we know it instinctively in India – Kali and Durga Mata ensure it. We need to see it more and more until the idea of a woman's courage is not relegated to labour and delivery, or the vigorous making of pasta or even carrying water across miles of dusty road.

If *Wonder Woman* is the modern girl child's first exposure to a woman warrior, then she will do the work that the Rani of Jhansi did for me. Let us free the warriors from the books in our attics and let them roam everywhere on our screens. Those who once were warriors were women too.

The strongest thing a man can do is cry.

Do you believe that? Or do you refute it with every fibre of your being? It's a Jay-Z quote. Does that change your opinion? I often hear of a person, generally a man, who waits until a swelling is the size of a grapefruit before going to a doctor. This is beyond my realm of experience. I live in the opposite land. The one where doctors are constantly telling me there's nothing wrong, they found nothing, the lupus is mild, the fever or tachycardia are not as bad as they have seen, always suppressing my apparent over-interest. The idea that a healthy person can disguise swellings on any part of their anatomy, or brush off concern, gives me pause. People call me brave. But isn't it braver to act nonchalant? Oh, this old grapefruit growing out of my neck? It's nothing. You should see the hernia beneath my jumper.

Or when men say they don't feel pain, or they don't take more than one painkiller. Why not? I ask. Because of the fear of addiction? They say, 'Painkillers don't touch my pain', hinting at a type of pain I could never imagine. I would like to invite these Trojans to step into my life – pick a page, any page, I want to invite them. And walk a little while in my shoes.

Nine years after my lymph node biopsy, I had the biopsy site surgically examined again. Nothing malignant was found, the culprit causing pockets of swelling was scar tissue. Nine years had not been long enough for the memory of pain from the old excavation to be forgotten. The nurse who offered me her hand to grip was not surprised by my tears but the doctor performing the procedure was unnerved. I was returned to the ward with no mention of painkillers, so that hours later, as my fellow patients were winding down to sleep, I was clawing the walls of my mind, loathe to think myself such a weakling.

My friend James rang. A surgeon himself, he diagnosed a lack of skill in the medic who had rooted around my lymph nodes and advised a dose of morphine for me. I was walking across the plank into shark infested waters by this point, and still unable to fully recognise that James was right.

I was too embarrassed to let him speak to the nurses on my behalf. In pain I might be, but still a feminist, I made the request myself. The tiniest dose. 2.5ml of Oromorph, swallowed easily. And I began to breathe easier, be calmed, become myself.

James prescribed morphine because I had suddenly burst into tears mid banal conversation, and in all our years of friendship, I had never done that.

'The strongest thing a man can do is cry,' says Jay-Z. What is the strongest thing a woman can do? Not cry? Laugh, then. But not too loudly. Not too obviously.

During a bout of kidney sepsis, I ended up on the Hepatology ward with two extraordinary patients. The first was a teenager who had attempted to commit suicide, not for the first time. I sat on the edge of her bed and talked her into laughter and possibilities. Between my bed by the window and hers by the nurses' station, was a woman drifting in and out of dementia. The nurses told us off for giggling, for talking too loudly – the patient between us needed her rest. Admonished, I slunk back to my bed. A few moments passed, lights out, silence. Then, a very particular fragrance arose between our beds. Someone was smoking a cigarette. I texted my new friend from beneath my bedsheet. 'No way! Is it you?' Of the three of us, I casually judged her for the rebel. 'No!' she texted back. And I knew she was laughing, quietly, as was I. Our crafty middle neighbour was burning the rules down.

What is courage? Is it playing the rebel? Is it stoic adherence to rules you hate, but comply with anyway?

How do we define courage? Is it the manly soldier bedecked with medals leaving for or returning from war? Or is it the uncomplaining, virtue signalling man who snaps, 'Stop making a fuss, woman!' when his wife suggests he visit the doctor?

Is courage sacrifice? Is it the doctor who conceals his or her personal suffering while dealing with a roster of suffering patients? Most people take great pride in carrying on even when they are sick. Hacking coughs, evident colds, 'Nothing stops me!' Meanwhile, the immune compromised person must stay home for double protection, feeling doubly shamed.

The lupus patient is always revving up to a battle that may never come. If it comes and we don't die, just linger on – are we still soldiers? We aren't fallen in a heroic way. We haven't won. And through it all, there is the deliberate instruction from society to 'man' this broken ship with élan. With courage. I don't mind being adjured to be courageous, to keep my chin up, to be grateful, to never give up, never lose hope – as long as my adjurers know the nature of the struggle against which that courage is measured.

There are still days when nausea overwhelms me even though I am no longer on weekly chemotherapy (Methotrexate) and the gaps between Rituximab doses are widening. It may be a combination of heavy-duty antibiotics combined with steroids and opiate based pain-killers making my head split from the desire to vomit out of a moving car. My mother would let me. She wouldn't care about the cars behind us. But when we pause by the railway line, and I do open the door to lean out, I somehow stop myself. Maybe the rush of cold air helps me gather myself. I hold the cells of my body together in a semblance of decency and rein myself back into the car. Maybe it's the absurdity of my mother's shock at my suggestion that I throw up into my soft pink bobble hat. *Not the hat! Just fling the car door open instead.*

Which do you think is worse? Which is better? Either way, the hat and the pavement survive. Is this my superpower? The ability to control my body's desire to violently express illness?

Six years after my three-month incarceration, I make a pilgrimage to the Infectious Diseases ward.

There is something eerie about the whole affair. Foolhardy. Like walking into a prison, voluntarily. My stomach does a tilt flop.

It's a Sunday. There have been other Sundays in here, but I was an in-patient then. Long quiet days when I could truly relax, when I was off duty from the sudden arrival of men in uniform, women in heels, marching purposefully towards my bed.

Some things remain the same. The scent of Burger King. Chips. Usual Sunday fare. On their weekend visits, my brothers could never resist, and even my father was partial to, a simple hamburger – no frills.

The absence of the suits is what makes the hospital sag a little with relief. You could almost believe there are no emergencies on Sundays.

Quiet deaths, yes. But some church-like sanctity pervades even these corridors.

I let myself into the old ward, walking behind a well-dressed member of staff. A medic? A pharmacist? The sense of being a criminal persists: a criminal on parole.

The nurse at the front desk looks at me seriously but doesn't stop me from walking past him and now I'm in. And I think I'm outside my old room, Bay 8. I recognize the basic layout. My heart is beating, a wild thing. What if time plays a trick on me and I fall back onto, into the bed that is inches away from me? I sit cautiously in the heft of the blue armchair that was always Dad's domain, even though it wrenched his back. All these years later, he still has residual strain.

Dear Shaista,
I am six years late in visiting you here in this room at this bed. I'm sorry.
I love you.

There is no one else in here. The walls are bare. No pictures of saints and prophets. The blue curtain is pulled back and a patient in the room opposite seems cheery enough. I don't remember being able to see other patients. I don't recall doors being left open.

The tea lady comes around. I ask her, partly out of genuine interest and partly to protect my shady wanderings, if she knows where Ana is. She doesn't know an Ana. The nurse in charge meanders over. Interested now.

The tea lady calls to someone over my shoulder. He, the cleaner, has been here longer than her. He might know Ana. I turn to him. Anna is on M4 now, he says. But the woman he is referring to is an English nurse, and my Ana was Portuguese, part of the housekeeping staff. I learn the history of the ward. It is no longer Infectious Diseases. It became Gastroenterology several years ago and most recently, Urology. This explains why I have been able to wander in so freely – Infectious Diseases requires masks and much greater care, stringent protocol. 'Do you work with her?' the tea lady asks. I tell the truth. I used to be a patient here.

The cleaner tilts his head and assesses me. *You're that girl who drew the picture?* Yes! I say. Although the person who drew *that* picture was my younger brother, Irfan. There were pictures all over my room but I know exactly which one he means. *Sai Baba of Shirdi*, he says. And I begin to cry.

The tea lady drifts away because I am now fully engaged in conversation with the cleaner. She doesn't see the tears. He leans back against the doorframe of an empty room and slightly averts his face. I wipe tears away. His name is Sundar. I remember him as he remembers me, my father, mother, brothers. 'So you finished your studies?' he asks. 'How are you now?'

Sundar and I talk a while. I tell him I am an aunty. 'And you?' he smiles. 'Still single?' Yup, I think, that's me. Still single. He was married then, six years ago, and now has two sons. He wants to be friends on Facebook. I say ok. We find each other on my phone.

Eventually, I leave. I step out, turn right and the sliding doors lead down the stairs to freedom, and the fields of gold beyond; I think of sitting outside on the steps but the sun drives me in again. I walk down the corridor, retracing my steps to the Jubilee Garden. Patients with giant indents of skull and tubing from various orifices are paraded past my bench in their wheelchairs. It's a Sunday. Visitors are here in droves. Well. Not exactly droves.

At the centre of the Jubilee Garden is a small stone statue. Carved into it are the words 'One Cannot Collect All The Beautiful Shells

On The Beach'. The words are a quote by Anne Morrow Lindbergh, although the statue does not mention her, only the man who cut the ribbon, and the date he did so. I think this: one does not return triumphant to a place of trauma. Sometimes, the place of trauma doesn't exist anymore. And sometimes, you are forced by circumstance to revisit the old haunts over and over again. The courage that is required of me involves me bringing myself to a place of terror, again. It's the second time that involves the act of courage. The second trabeculectomy, knowing the first felt like shards of glass crunching into and across my cornea. The second cycle of Diamox, remembering the sensation of spiders crawling all over my flesh. Having walked through the memory of the first, and embodied the raw newness of it, I must walk towards it again.

This is not a book about being a warrior. This book is about resistance. Living is an act of resistance. Living past death and through a half-life into a full life is an act of resistance. That is my personal act of courage. I resist prevailing attitudes about sickness, about women, about art and writing, about success and failure, even about vulnerability and strength. I resist the metaphor and mythology imposed upon the sick and look only to connect.

ONLY CONNECT

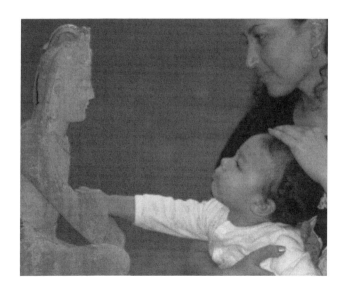

The Year of Yes

I wish I had said yes, beloved,
when you asked me out to walk

among the leaves,
the turning leaves,

you were offering me the sound of dreams
and I turned you down, politely.

Not today, I smiled.
Perhaps, maybe, tomorrow?

But I wish I had said yes, beloved,
I wish we had shared this light.

Next time don't ask, just take me!
Order me to dress.

I am going to need your help, beloved,
to begin the year of yes.

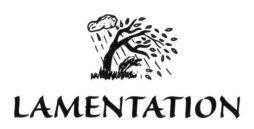

LAMENTATION

Your house is on fire.

'Don't worry about it,' says the fireman. 'I am putting it out.'

'I will do my best,' he amends.

You ask: 'But what about all the things I will lose in the fire?'

Ah. Those. The fireman and the doctor know nothing about those. What is lost is yours to mourn in private.

Let us talk about it, then. The thing we avoid. The thing called grief that must be pushed aside at all possible cost. Because how would you get your work done? How would you feed the children and make the bills go away?

It can happen in childhood, defining the rest of adulthood to come. Your father or mother, the person you hero worship, leaves you. It can happen late in life, when your grown daughter or son dies, leaving you long before they were meant to. They were never meant to leave you.

Or it happens the day you are diagnosed with a tumour.

We come up with clichés like 'life is too short' but we are overwhelmed by the longitude of a single day, exhausted by the end of a single year because of the accumulation of moments, memories.

We grieve. And we pretend not to.

But what power there is in sharing grief. I don't see the revelation as weakness. Ruby Wax revealed to us in her episode of 'Who Do You Think You Are?' that if her mother had cried, just once, and shown the inner face of her sorrow at bearing witness to Kristallnacht, the terrible Night of Broken Glass, in November 1938, when thousands of Jewish-owned stores and synagogues were smashed with sledgehammers, Wax could have forgiven her the rest.

We make up stories about ourselves and others when the truth remains hidden. We know no other way. Better to share the real story, I think. The truth is so much easier to forgive in the end.

Lupus is not a degenerative illness. But it is cumulative. I went into hospital as a ten-year old, under the protective aegis of my father. I knew no fear then. At least none that I recall. Being the Head of the Radiology Department meant that Dad was a focal point for other consultants who would drop in on him in his ground floor rooms and pick his diagnostic brain over fluorescent X rays. He inspired respect but beyond respect, he did that other mysterious thing that only some human beings are able to do. He made people laugh. What magical element makes us laugh? Makes us make others laugh? We try not to decode this too deeply, so essential an ingredient is this alchemy.

Doctors have always had access to humour. It is almost taken for granted that a doctor will have a sense of the absurd sitting alongside the profound. For a patient, dealing in absurdities is not the crux of this way of life. It can be dangerous, because of the unequal distribution of power. A patient reveals their distress. The doctor asks, 'Have you talked to anyone about this?' The doctor is referring to a professional therapist. The patient thinks, 'But I *am* talking to someone, right now. You.'

Doctors can be described as non-patients. But they can be patients too. There is a potential to connect in fellowship, but doctors rarely reveal their personal vulnerabilities. Is it because they are professionally bound not to? Why? Because it would blur boundaries? Who designs the boundaries? Would a doctor lose power if she shared her own experience with illness? I believe she would gain connection.

A patient could write a Kafkaesque or Beckettian piece on bureaucracy in the system – plenty of material for absurdity there – but the lived experience of being at the receiving end of failed, inexplicable bureaucracy is the desire to die. Mostly there is a 'keep your head down, don't disturb the status quo, be grateful' approach to any aspect of your life that involves bureaucracy. At the hospital, you are not at home. There have been several occasions when I have forgotten this simple fact and after a long stay, bought into the fantasy of the room being my room, the bed being my bed. And on my day of departure, I have attachment issues that only fellow inmates might appreciate.

Hospitals are places of edges. No exchange between staff and sufferer is ever quite right. Friendliness can be misconstrued or mis-judged and the rest is a slow or sudden dehumanisation. Kindness becomes so extraordinarily precious that it is equally destroying; it leaves you more vulnerable than ever to the next abrasion or invasion. Patients are not supposed to give doctors gifts, but we don't know this to be a clear, unbreakable rule. The clearest social rule, taught in childhood, is to thank people who have helped you. In India, doctors are always given boxes of sweetmeats or invitations to weddings. The gift is to honour and be honoured. Do the gifts constitute bribery? What is being solicited? Further kindness? Continued compassion?

What I would love more than anything is for there to be a democratic understanding between medics and patients. The ideal human interaction is one where needs are met equally. I am constantly striving towards equality, towards a sense of fairness for our place in the world. One way into such progress is through being useful, but there is a fine line between being useful and being used. A chronic illness patient is regularly subjected to being used within the context of being useful – at some nebulous future point. 'We are doing this for you,' say the researchers and laboratory technicians as they draw more blood, extract more marrow, ask more questions about your race, age, pregnancy status. What they mean is, 'This will all help you someday, but right now, it will really help me in my career.'

When campylobacter entered my bloodstream some years ago, the Infectious Diseases team asked me to sign a consent form for my case to be written up as a paper. I signed willingly because I had been led to believe that the team wanted to collaborate with me. My gratified ego gave consent. Later, when I heard nothing further from the team, I realised I had been seduced by the possibility of intellectual equality into giving my consent. Later still, it occurred to me that I had never been asked for my signed consent before, which meant that in my early years of medical celebrity, I must surely have been written up without permission. Where is the rule book on intellectual medical consent?

In the summer of 1998, when I was about to turn twenty, I had begun to display disturbing signs of cerebral disease: photophobia, involuntary movements, facial dysesthesia. The rheumatologists requested a second opinion with a consultant ophthalmologist (Dr. Meyer, who immediately diagnosed glaucoma) but not before one last trauma. Here is a diary entry from that summer:

August 11, 1998

Dr. C, one of the consultants, thinks I definitely have cerebral lupus, but the whole team is not in agreement. To satisfy some of them, they want to do another spinal tap.

Two weeks ago, I begged Dr. G to do the first tap because I trusted him completely. He refused. He had already promised the job to two junior doctors. One of them missed and hit a nerve. In my spine. You don't die from pain, however much you may want to. I am learning this. I think I floated somewhere because I can see myself lying on my front, the needle in my back, my fingers curled into the sheets, one word on my tongue. Ma.

I have refused a second lumbar puncture.

I look back at the girl lying face down on the bed with two junior doctors 'having a go' at my spine, not believing them when they said they would go away if I wanted them to, because I knew they would come back; they had to get the fluid; somebody always 'has to' do something to you in hospital because somebody else said so. As though everyone is following a central head that is controlling the rest of the staff like puppets and they are the helpless ones, not us. Later, I will read Dr. C's words in my notes:

She will not allow a repeat LP and that seems reasonable.

The gulf between a medic's language and ours could not be greater. No matter what I suffer, their notes will always tell a very different tale. A reasonable one.

Anger still chokes me from time to time because experimental treatment is still the name of the game. *Let's try this and see how we go. Let's take this away and see how you fare.* The dynamic tension of doctors not knowing very much about lupus and yet requiring the patient to be submissive and co-operative, is evident in *The Habit of Being*, the collected letters of Flannery O'Connor, who was twenty-five when she was diagnosed with lupus. She hated the disease because it interfered with her writing, but she wrote right up until her death on August 3, 1964. She was thirty-nine when she died. Allowing for her commentary on Catholicism and her indifference to the civil rights movement, her letters are a masterclass in wit, and a gracious acceptance of her reality. Here is an example:

> *You have to be very careful what you say to or show doctors. Remove any traces of imagination or anything not 20-20 facts. I waddn't born yesterday… I don't get any information out of them that I particularly understand but then I'd have to study medicine if I wanted to keep up with myself. I don't know if I'm making progress or if there's any to be made. Let's hope they are learning something anyhow.*

My hospital, Addenbrooke's, is a teaching hospital. The professors and consultants I meet are generally academics, in some capacity attached to the University of Cambridge. Research can come before humanity. Fascination with a subject can make some forget there are actual lives at stake in the here and now. In 1995, Margaret Edson detailed this beautifully in her scathing play 'Wit', which follows the life of an English professor dying of ovarian cancer. *What we have come to think of as me*, she writes, *is in fact just the specimen jar, just the dust jacket, just the white piece of paper that bears the little black marks.*

Words bother me as a writer, and I was a writer long before the disease clawed into me. When doctors throw words at me – phrases, received jargon and, most of all, analogy – pincers shoot out of me. 'What did you mean by that?' I challenge. 'Why did you say that?' It isn't that I intend to be difficult or troublesome, but language is the landscape I draw meaning from. I need things to be clear, or if that is impossible, then at least trustworthy. Words leave marks and indents.

'Let me try explaining lupus to you the way I see it,' said a GP, intending camaraderie. 'You are rotting, and fast. The only thing in some measure controlling the speed of rotting are the drugs you are on. Stop them, or try to tinker with them, and...'

A menacing pause.

No need for it, really. I was stuck on 'rotting'. 'Rotting' has stuck on me, a little barnacle I cannot shake off, though a decade or more has passed.

⌒

Soon after the Molteno implant surgery, I brought myself into A&E, my eye in sharp discomfort. Keith was unfortunately not available that day, so another ophthalmologist took a look. He found the suture that was irritating my eyelid and said he would cut it. He proceeded with no anaesthesia. I finally had to beg him to stop, through tears. He agreed to. My eye was bruised and swollen. Later, as I was standing near the door with Mum, he came by and said, 'Are you still crying?'

Two days later, when I returned, Keith was very surprised that his colleague had not used anaesthetic drops. He bathed my eye into numbness and within a minute had skillfully extracted five sutures. It felt peaceful having him attend to my eye while it rained and cool breezed outside. I acknowledged the difference in skill between the two doctors, but also in compassion. Keith somehow always knew when not to banter.

Keith didn't have a monopoly on kindness. Once, after a particularly grim appointment about my eyes with Dr. Meyer, I stopped by a favourite window and wept. Philip, one of the young ophthalmic registrars, was walking up from the opposite direction. He made a joke about me choosing an interesting spot for a weep. I appreciated his intention to make me smile because in every encounter with me he had been kind and gentlemanly. I turned up the corners of my mouth. Batted back a feeble retort.

Sometimes I have the energy for wit, and sometimes not. Sometimes it is engaging and amusing, and elicits a smile, a retort, a small human exchange. Nothing memorable. It simply passes the time in a way bearable to the spirit. Other times, it is inappropriate, but there is no way to tell. I never know if someone is going to misuse the banter and slip, beneath my frail veneer, a careless dagger.

The difficult patient is so called because she demands visibility. She demands a level of humanity that is greater than protocol sees fit. Protocol leaves little or no room for individual choices of kindness and compassion, or wisdom. Protocol enables a doctor to make notes about a patient that would make the patient cringe with embarrassment.

I had been struggling with a tooth infection some years ago. The first dentist I saw temporarily fixed the broken molar and sent me off with this Parthian shot: 'You can die from a tooth infection.' Who needs enemies? By the time a different dentist advised a tooth extraction, 'you can die from a tooth infection' had worked its way into the root of me where fear and courage have their daily tussle. I am on chemotherapy, I have an unpredictable illness; fear was winning, and I openly shared my anxiety with the second dentist. I wanted her to reassure me, but she opted for honesty: 'I'm not sure I'll be able to take the whole tooth out. You may need to go to a dental hospital.' I agreed to the referral. It seemed sensible. I waited a month. No word. I rang the dental hospital only to be informed by a lovely receptionist that my referral had been triaged to my main hospital, because the dentist had written *This patient is very nervous and very scared of treatment* in her notes. The dental hospital was, understandably, reluctant to take on such a liability. *This patient is very nervous and very scared of treatment* is now available online for every member of the NHS staff to see. No context provided about why the patient had expressed anxiety.

Eventually, I was seen by the oral surgery team at the hospital. The young female trainee smiled at me and I was comforted. She attempted the extraction but failed to remove my tooth. Behind her, a man rose from his chair. He was the oral surgeon. He was a large man. He struggled to remove my tooth. I thought he would break my jaw with his efforts. My heart tried to tear itself free. There were windows in front of me. I wanted wings. I needed flight. He could sense my terror. He told me I needed to raise my hand if I wanted him to stop. He could not concentrate on both my mouth and the possibilities of my unmoving hand. I didn't raise my hand. Later, I wished I had. I didn't cry tears, but something wept inside me, in the place where I am tired of things being done to me for my own good. I wanted my tooth back. I want my sight back. I want my home back.

The second time I had a tooth extracted, the dentist showed me her archaeological findings. She did ask first. I have the image now in my head. I can piece together the experience of what I was feeling as she went to work with tools above my face, and the reality of what she did. What she took out of my body and laid upon a tray. Is it better to see or not see? Can what has been seen be unseen? A doctor offers: would you like to keep your appendix? The remains of a loved one? You have to decide if you'd like to keep the ashes of your loved one near. Or let go.

Which is worse? Seeing the real or imagining the unseen?

I didn't know the root of a tooth was so big. The size of an adult nail. I can feel the missing gap with my tongue inside and with my fingers outside, along my jaw.

We hate loss. We don't want to learn spiritual lessons at the cost of loss. We want it all. Why can't we have it all? We'd be happy then, all of us, wouldn't we?

There are other ways to deal with a tooth extraction than an elegiac response. My grandmother devoured a pork chop the same evening she had her tooth removed. Mouth bloody? Socket sore? Sure, but pass up a pork chop? Not Vera. Mind you, had the meal that evening not appealed to her, she would have been just as capable of pulling a sad face and blaming a sore socket and a mouth full of blood for her sudden loss of appetite. '*Ghanu dukhech, dikra,*' she would have said. It hurts too much, my child.

When you consider yourself an intelligent woman, you cannot contain the prideful need to demand transparency. 'Tell me everything,' you try to convey, but tears blur your martial spirit after the first brutalities, your face gives away too much of your frailty and suddenly, you just want to be loved and told everything will be alright. But it is too late. You already asked to be told the truth.

Honesty. Do you think it is overrated? Or underrated? I have a fluid relationship with honesty in my medical life as I suspect most doctors do. No doctor can achieve the perfect balance with a patient. Given time, a patient's harsh first assessment of a doctor's character and manner can soften and even completely change. But time is generally not the patient's friend.

Nor is it the doctor's friend; often, doctors forget the significance of the seemingly basic courtesy of introducing themselves before they dive into examining, diagnosing or prescribing you medication. There is something powerful and essential about that moment of introduction, about a handshake. A moment of contact that exactly parallels a social encounter, reminding both parties there is a human element here. We could have met outside of the domain of white beds and blue paper curtains. We still might. Today, it sounds almost challenging to ask a doctor to repeat or spell their name, if their name is hard to catch. As though you are trying to catch them out, or keep the name for later, in case of trouble. And yet *our* names are inscribed on every piece of paper along with our ages, addresses and the intricacies of our bodily fluids.

Michael, my fellow patient on Rituximab, tells me he does not respond to doctors who ask him questions while looking at their screen. He waits until the doctors swivel their heads around, probably checking whether Michael has heard them, or perhaps annoyed that the answer wasn't delivered promptly enough.

While we talk, a nurse painstakingly peels off the tape that secures his IV tube to his arm. Michael cuts his eyes at me. 'The doctors just rip it off,' he says. 'And then they look at me. They like to see the pain.' I think he is joking when he says this. But I can't be sure.

Nowadays, I am older than the medical students who examine or question me and it is rare for me to be caught off guard by insensitivity; I am developing a shield of detached, humorous armour. I like to think of my detached humour as a form of compassion to myself, and others; years of succumbing to sensitivity leaves you with an unbalanced feeling. With time, my perspective has shifted from wanting to erase myself, to wanting to make myself visible, to finally, trying to be just as visible as is bearable to my witness. In other words, trying to see and be seen in equal measure.

When my infusion tube gets blocked from time to time on the infusion bay, a nurse prepares a syringe of saline and tries to push some saline through. I hold my breath while my mind prepares itself for unknown quantities of pain. She holds the syringe. She can push at any rate or any strength; I have no control. I could use words like *Stop! Don't!* But I rarely call halt. Or how would anything ever move forward? If I could have called halt, I would have done so a very long time ago, when I was seven and my eyes first began losing focus, and there was nothing I could do, nothing my parents could do, to stop the advancing, retreating dance of seeing differently.

THE MONKEY'S PAW

When I was at school in India, I acted in a play called *The Monkey's Paw*, based on a supernatural short story written by W. W. Jacobs in 1902.

I played Mrs White, who, along with her husband, becomes the new inheritor of a mummified monkey's paw imbued with the power to grant three wishes. The wishes, however, come with a price for interfering with fate. Ignoring the post-colonial ironies of Indian school children playing a British family destroyed by Indian sorcery, I inherited something of that fateful thinking.

Be careful what you wish for.

We aren't supposed to want more than one thing. We aren't supposed to ask for more than one thing. We are taught to concentrate on one prayer at a time. After all, how can you be faithful and fickle at the same time? I have taught myself to follow this tradition: ask for health, and I might be given it. But I want to be a writer. A real writer. So then, I must give up on good health. What about love? I can't have it all? So then, not the health, and not the ever after love. I'll take the writing. I'll take the creations that emerge from the tips of my fingers. Thought to words.

What do you want to be when you grow up? I never said anything about a man. Or marriage. And I knew too little about illness to be concerned with health. I knew enough about the kind of love that matters. I was already loved. I am loved still, in the same way, by the same hearts that loved me then.

.

In the back of the car one day, either in Singapore, or England, or Portugal, Rafael muses out loud: 'Aunty Shai hasn't got any children.'

'I haven't,' I agree.

'Because you don't have a husband, Aunty Shai. Who is going to be your husband?'

Raf worries about my marital status.

'I don't know, Scruffs. I don't know,' I say, unable to provide comfort.

Dear husband,

I am so sorry I lost two teeth and a spleen along the way, but I still have two kidneys, which is actually an achievement for twenty years of serious lupus activity. My toes were a mess of infection and vasculitis back when I was nineteen, but they are all present and correct today. Pretty too, when pretty is called for.

Will that do?

Is it better to lose parts of our bodies after marriage or before we even have a chance to be beautiful, once upon a time, in a young lover's dream?

I'll never know at this rate. The verdict according to some is that youth is no longer mine to claim. 'You're not young anymore,' said a GP to me, clarifying this for herself after glancing at my birth date on the computer screen. I hadn't asked for her opinion on the matter, but I was given it anyway.

I disliked being asked my age between twenty-five and thirty-five. My questioner would assume I was young enough to be asked my age, and upon the number being revealed, surprise would turn to pity.

Surprise because I was clearly bearing up well under the burden of old age. Pity upon further questioning revealing no husband and no children. And then the comforting pat. 'You'll find someone. I'm sure the right one will come along. You can still have children.'

In my thirty-fifth year, both my sisters-in-law became pregnant, and were due to deliver three baby girls within weeks of each other. In order to be with them on their baby journey, I followed their progress through a website called BabyCentre. They were, naturally, able to put their own names into the registration page and follow their actual pregnancy to birth process; me, I put in my name, and one day I received this happy, congratulatory email:

> 'Hello Shaista,
> Any day now, you'll be a mum! Let's hope you won't have to wait too much longer for the big event. And try not to worry if it feels like your baby's staying firmly put. Most babies arrive later than their due date. Turn these last few days to good use. Go over your birth plan with your partner, to make sure you've covered everything. You may start to feel differently about earlier decisions now the prospect of labour and birth is becoming very real. Spend some special time with your partner, or, if you have older children, enjoy these days with them. You'll be glad you did once your baby comes.'

It was a little weird.

It doesn't break my heart every day. I am not wandering around with an open wound every time thoughts of other women's pregnancies occur. I entered into the dialogue with my sisters readily and with enthusiasm. These will be my nieces, I thought. I am connected. And will always be someone special to them.

Nor is this the end of my life. Despite several stages along the road when I have been at a possible end, the battle has so far proven miraculously in my favour. I may yet survive a while longer, but the quality of that life is the heart of the matter.

'Any chance you could be pregnant?'
I have been asked this question since I was eighteen and first diagnosed with lupus. It is a routine question asked by nurses, GPs, anesthetists. It is a box on a checklist that needs to be crossed or ticked because modern medicine was not designed for the female body; toxic medications were not trialed on women and therefore did not take fertility into account.

Through most of my illness, my mother has accompanied me during A&E consultations. Often, the person asking me this question flicks a look across at my mother, as though to suggest that my answer might be different if she were absent from the room. Over the years, I have been embarrassed, amused, saddened and recently, angered, when a male doctor overrode my clear negative response with, 'Let's just do a pregnancy test anyway', as though I might be confused, or, since my mother was present, lying.

'At least you can give the baby back!'
Why do people tell me this, as though it is the ultimate joy of an aunt? How is the best thing about being an aunt giving the baby back? Where does this saying come from? The best thing about being an aunt is in the sharing of holding the baby together, of sharing in the parent-approved rearing of the children we are so fortunate to love in unqualified measures. There is no giving back because there is no taking away.

During my year of the double sister pregnancy, a YouTube documentary about the life of the Irish novelist, Maeve Binchy, serendipitously found its way to me. When her mother died of cancer in 1968,

Binchy moved back to the family home in Dalkey, Dublin. When her father died in 1971, Binchy was thirty-two, and she expected to lead a life of spinsterhood. When she fell in love and married Gordon Snell, the British author of children's literature, in 1977, their happiness was only marred by the discovery that they couldn't have children. Binchy's words gave me great strength:

> *I think it's a lovely thing if you know somebody who has no children, to share your children with them, from an early age, and let them see the bad as well as the good. Not just only the bits where they have success of graduation, or engagement parties or anything like that, or birthdays. Let them be involved in the bad bits as well.*

It is my good fortune that I am an aunt who gets to see 'the bad bits as well'.

Aunty Shai. How did this happen? How am I suddenly picturing myself at sixty-three just so I can picture my nephew at thirty? I age myself ruthlessly, just so I can imagine the kind of teenagers they will one day be. Will they love me then as they love me now, calling out my name first thing in the morning and last thing at night? 'Shai! Shai! Shai! Shai!'

When he was three years old, Rafael used to begin every conversation with, 'Tell me a story, Aunty Shai' and no other lead in. Irfan would prompt his single-minded son, 'Don't you want to say *hello, how are you, Aunty Shai? How was your weekend?*'

'No,' was the short, sturdy response.

And on its heels, swift and sure, 'Tell me a story, Aunty Shai.' There were no exclamation points at the end of his demand. There was nothing wheedling about his request. It was, in a way, the first line of the story to come. Instead of 'Once upon a time', Raf began with, 'Tell me a story'.

Of late, when faced with the bald truth of the story of my age, my interlocutor doesn't want to give me false hope. There was still hope at thirty-five, but now there remains only the comforting pat.

Would they pity me more if they knew I have a simple wedding planned out, down to all essential details?

Where: Our garden.

What I'll wear: Mum's wedding sari (white, with embroidered gold stars), flower crowns for me, Bella, Eva and Ellie. Raf will be the ring bearer.

To whom? This alone is the unresolved, unseeable, unknowable mystery.

Should I fix the date of my wedding and trust the person will come as ultra-Orthodox, Hasidic, Michal does, in Rama Burshtein's romantic comedy *Through The Wall?* Michal wills herself to believe that if she is good, and has faith, a husband will appear in time for the pre-booked wedding date of the eighth night of Chanukah. Or maybe I could have the marriage ceremony sans person? Just me marrying air, earth and sky. Surrounded by love. Married, by threads of love, to those I love.

The greatest non-marital adventure I am on, is being available to love and be loved without a fixed fulcrum. I imagine once beringed, the centre of your gravity shifts and The Person, Your Person, becomes your personal sun. And you the moon. Or you the moon, and they the earth. Metaphorical language always lands me in confusion.

The language of the spirit is no clearer. At nineteen, I had my first near-death experience. I saw the light, in the corner of my hospital room. I saw the threads that connected me to those who had gone before – the grandfather I had known and the one I never knew. The aunt and grandmother I had never met. The figures felt real but the decision to stay or join them was mine alone to make. In the balance, another vision offered itself. Myself, with a flower crown. A wedding. A joyful celebration. Surely mine? But I have lived long enough past that night to have seen my brothers married in just such a way – garlands of flowers, rice thrown, my mother reciting Avestan prayers.

I think about it sometimes. At the length of time I have had to prepare for the entrance of a person to whom I may bind myself. I don't know how I will ever learn to share with another human being a body that has been so consistently scrutinised in the most unromantic of ways. There is no portion of me that this disease has not already laid claim to like some hungry ghost, devouring me with more thoroughness than any corporeal lover. How will I allow myself to believe this flesh is not simply laboratory material? Blood, marrow, sclera, cornea, derma. I am more familiar with the original Latinate words, clinical in their usage today. Who will translate the clinician's dictionary of jargon into words of poetry and passion? Can it be done?

I know what it is to be viewed by cold, impersonal eyes, and cold, impersonal scopes. I remember noticing a young doctor's shoes. He was a very natty dresser. His shirt, pink, beautifully ironed. But it was his shoes I stared at the most. They were shiny, but not obtrusively so. They were a mark of expense. I learned later he was a Cambridge graduate. He didn't seem to see me at all. There was a problem with my drug chart. I was reacting badly to a prescribed level, and he, the doctor on call, arrived to adjust it. He neither introduced himself, nor favoured me with more than a cursory glance. He was all business and busyness. I preoccupied myself with his pretty shoes, so I didn't have to feel less human than I already did.

Sometimes the interaction between a male doctor and his female patient can bear resemblance to a brief flirtation. But there will always be a rather brutal end to that flirtation. During one of my shorter admissions, a woman was whisked in by ambulance after a fall. She had none of her home comforts with her, not her hairbrush nor her prescription glasses. When the consultant arrived, he was all charm. He oozed the intelligence of another Cambridge man, an academic as much as a clinician. He coaxed her out of her chair (he had not witnessed the great difficulty with which she had climbed into it, earlier that morning) and back into her dreaded bed. Dreaded because of the blood that had pooled onto her pillow from the gashes on the back of her scalp. But she really had no choice, and I did mention the fluidity of his charm.

She lay subservient to his touch as he manipulated this joint and that. Needing to check her feet, he requested permission to remove her socks. He removed her socks. He completed his examination and then he departed, all cheer, almost whistling. There was silence. And then she spoke aloud, to me, to the listening world to which she really belonged – the sockless, the disempowered. 'They come. They take off your socks. And then they leave. Never occurs to them. To put. Your socks. Back on!'

With movements fractured by a bruising pain I could only guess at, she drew on courage I didn't have to guess at, and inch by inch worked her body over to her side. At which point I was up, her socks in my hand, bent at her feet, ready for each foot. She let me. After all, we had just laughed together. We were comrades in a bloody sport. Faceless, because our faces will not be remembered by the doctors who forget to put our socks back on, nor even by each other. I could not describe her face to you now, nor, I doubt, would she remember mine. Either way, we won't be tested on this.

When doctors fail on their face recognition abilities, it feels personal. When I was nineteen, the doctor who ignored my plea to do a spinal tap himself, was still my favourite, my confidante, at the end of my admission. One day, soon after, when I returned for an outpatient appointment, I saw him in the concourse. He was walking towards me with a medical colleague. My face lit up. My mouth half opened in greeting. He walked past me. Perhaps he never saw me. Perhaps he did.

I am not speaking of love anymore. I am speaking of men. Of male doctors. And that is not the same thing. Except that it would be disingenuous to pretend that the one never has anything to do with the other. But even when I did read Mills & Boon, I cannot recall doctor-patient trysts. Only doctor-nurse trysts. And those were trying enough to imagine since my father was a doctor and even *my* imagination stopped short of any unprofessional scenarios.

How will it happen? When will it happen? Where will it happen? I had bare shoulders and hibiscus in my hair on Nikoi Island to offer someone, even the Gold Coast, giggling at skippy kangaroos. I had the scent of lemons on my skin in Limone on the shore of Lake Garda to offer, and even poetry in Prague, by moonlight. There was a petite blond-haired violinist who played a scintillating piece of Dvořák aimed directly at me. You think I am being vain, but there were only three of us in the audience; one was his grandfather and the other my travelling companion. She didn't begrudge me the attention. He was half her height and with a rabbit-caught-in-the-headlights look about him. Still, the Dvořák was delicious.

I am capable of imagining myself the muse of a talented director or conductor or worthy academic. Plucked from obscurity by the way my shadow falls across a courtyard. Being the writer and director of my imaginary scripts, I include sparkling dialogue; I am witty even when I don't mean to be. A vulnerable, tragi-comic figure.

But even into this romance, controlled in its entirety by my mind, some vestiges of reality creep in. I know love is possible at any age or stage of human existence, but the romance of our international movie and musical worlds rests heavily upon energy. Midway through my scripted drama, I have tired myself out with sparkle and wit. Enough! I think, turning over in my bed, gathering up a handful of sheet or biting savagely into the side of a pillow. It's not real.

This inability to move forward with my internal script is partly a result of the lack of visual representation of sexuality with disability. Romance braided in with cancer has been accepted into the canon, because the roles are played by physically perfect film stars who we know are not ill in reality. Tom Hanks himself did not have AIDS in *Philadelphia*. We are asked to suspend belief for an hour and a half and we do so. We are not being asked to believe that sweeping acts of romance are occurring between a person who is really sick and their healthy lover. And there usually is a healthy lover, male or female, in the cinematic narrative. *Love and Drugs* comes closest to acknowledging some of the complications of shame, guilt and pride that inform such relationships. There was a perfect note struck by Richard Curtis in *Notting Hill* between the characters Max and Bella, with Bella's wheelchair written in and out of significance, according to the needs of the human being in the chair, rising to meet the story. And I felt these echoes of understanding in Guillermo del Toro's *The Shape of Water*, but here, understanding is achieved through the fictional being of an amphibian sea-monster. For those of us longing for more accurate representations, the film canon falls woefully short.

I know this much about love: when it does happen, even in its least perfect form, it is real. And I can only hope that when the time comes, if it comes, life will supply the energy I need to meet my fellow partner in dance. Perhaps not step for step, but enough. Enough.

What you don't know when it all begins, is how much you will end up loving yourself, in spite of yourself. In spite of the lupus. Not *my*

lupus. I didn't name this thing. I don't have to claim it to love myself.
And I do love myself because I keep myself company through it all. I
am the friend in the in-between hours. I am the first thing I wake up to.
My voice, in my head. I amuse myself with my own chatter.

I talk to myself. Is this a form of madness?

It is the most companionable thing. It never feels like a monologue.
It feels like I am talking to an extremely interested listener, who doesn't
interrupt my stream of consciousness.

I like the sound of my own voice when nobody is listening. Trees
don't seem to mind. Birds and animals hear me from miles off, but they
are listening for the language my feet speak or the rustle of my coat.

I'd like to put this down to the writing of memoir, of recording
myself out of and inside real time. But I have always enjoyed conversations with myself for as long as I have had language. Who better to talk
to than myself? I know exactly what interests me, and which thought
strand to investigate. I meander but never mind the meandering. I have
always enjoyed my brain, its capacity for thought and word, and even
though I spend more hours alone than in company, I still feel lonely for
myself when in company. It is peaceful being me, with me.

I can feel this peaceful with Mum, but no one else. With everyone
else, there is always an element of performance to keep the story going.
The story of courage, witticism and positivity. Or even of truth telling
but telling it well. Making the suffering concise, balanced. Above all,
don't be boring. Because there is nothing duller than talking health.
Good, bad or indifferent.

Or perhaps it is as simple as knowing my mother loves me, uncon-
ditionally. I never have to ask *do you love me?* Except, of course, I do.
Regularly. Followed by *but why? Give me reasons. Be specific.* She never
indulges me. 'I just do,' she says, ending the conversation and satisfying
me, at one and the same time.

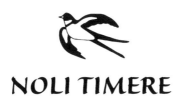

NOLI TIMERE

At Seamus Heaney's memorial service, Michael Heaney shared with us the last text message his father sent his mother.

Two words, in Latin. *Noli timere*. Be not afeared. Let nothing affright thee. Seamus Heaney was an alchemist transforming fear into fearlessness.

My own alchemist lives in the room down the corridor from mine. Sometimes we WhatsApp each other from our rooms. Other times, receiving his message of fearlessness involves the following exercise.

It starts with me moseying down the corridor to Dad's room. I open the door and find him on the floor, contorted into one of his yogic positions.

I sit in his vacant chair and put my head in my hands.

'Dad,' I croak.

'Yes?'

I sigh. Then huff out, 'What are you doing?'

'Just my exercises.'

Just. Blind and eighty-four, there is no *just* about this. This is will-power. The inspirational, if-I-put-it-on-YouTube-would-go-viral kind of *just*.

I slink lower into his chair.

'Have you done yours?' comes the muffled question from the inside of a cheek smushed to carpet.

'No,' I gripe, as though I am twelve and being asked if I've done extra maths homework (which we used to do for our tuition teacher Mr Imdad, a delightful man with the almost impossible task of making maths as delightful as he himself was).

By this point, Dad has curved himself out into bow pose, toes to the back of his head. *Dhanurasana*, if you know your Sanskrit. To strengthen the back.

I can't take it anymore. 'I'm off, Pops,' I offer his concentrated form. And weasel away before the guilt of witnessing more inspiration overwhelms me.

We will meet later anyway, somewhere along that corridor between my room and his. 'Hello,' I'll say. 'It's you,' he'll say. I might slip my hand into his to shake it. He might take my pulse. We are always taking each other's pulse. Still alive? Still alive. And what more can either of us ask of each other, when being alive and together is the sweetest fruit we have to offer?

The third wheel in our Beckettian routine is nestled somewhere in one of the rooms, writing, painting, contemplating cooking or attending to the laundry. Or fighting to save a withered plant from an unnecessary grave. The green fingered one who keeps the others alive in a more practical way than terse pulse taking and jerky, dislocated humour.

In the eye clinic, a woman once told me that she was glad when she finally went blind. The pain and obfuscation of her eye disease had been worse than the finality of total vision loss. I listened and accepted this was the case for her. I have never forgotten her words. They come back to haunt me on my worst eye days. And I wonder, do I feel the same?

I don't. I would take the pain and unfocused frustration every day over the darkness. Let me have light for as long as I can.

Everything passes, they say.
Things can always be worse, I think.

This is my motto:
Get a grip.
Get a grip, Shaista.

I don't say it unkindly. And usually, it works.

This is what I know: that I have nothing to offer you. If death came for me, you would acknowledge I had suffered enough and let me go. If death came for you or the one you love, what good am I and my suffering? Grief is still the one place no one can fight to enter without permission. If you found your way to Joan Didion's *The Year of Magical Thinking* and she spoke to you, loss to loss, it was a private conversation. If I sent you Didion, would that not be an intrusion? Who am I to send you a book on grief when you are grieving not Didion's husband or her daughter but your own beloved?

With illness, no such intrusion is considered. With illness, you will constantly be sent books on illness and recovery, on how to be better and how to be sick. But although you may feel obliged to read these books you will always want to write your own book, tell your own story, because that is what is being drowned out by the other books being sent your way. In the end, you may write your own book. And it will be described as catharsis. Because no one can believe you would want to write the truth of your experience for any other purpose than to extinguish it like a ghost squelched by lamplight. I don't write for catharsis. I write to tell the truth of my life. I was here. I wrote. And I carried on living, just the same. With all those truths intact.

Growing older has given me some measure of insight, but even age cannot prepare you for the energy of the evangelical. One of the greatest joys in my life occurred in the summer of 2012, when I was able to attend a week's retreat at Plum Village, the hermitage home of Thich Nhât Hanh. I had been practicing mindfulness in Thây's style of engaged Buddhism since 2005, the year of the Molteno operation and the corneal ulcer, but never imagined I would fulfill my dream of walking between plum trees in the Dordogne to the sound of the great bell. In between walking and eating meditation, there were talks given by Thây, and on a rare occasion, time to sit at the feet of Sister Chân Không, a peace activist equally responsible for the global work of the Order of Interbeing. Sister Chân Không was inviting us to share our stories of grief. I confided something of my long life with illness and the toll of losses such a life invariably bestows upon us. In the middle of my telling, a woman to my left interrupted to inform me that she had the answer to my problem. 'NLP,' she said. She described it briefly and told me she would speak to me later in more detail. Sister Chân Không looked at both of us, no doubt pleased that the young people were helping each other. I couldn't think clearly beyond knowing my only chance of hearing the personalised wisdom of one of the most extraordinary Venerable nuns had just disappeared. Outside the hall, the woman hurried up to me, and perhaps she offered a contact address, perhaps not. I only remember trying to explain to her that grief was normal, that I hadn't been looking for a solution to a problem. I had simply been sharing my story.

How often do you cry? I remember the first time I saw my mother cry. My great-aunt Khorshed had rung with news of my great-grandmother Tehmina's death. I'm not sure I recall my mother crying at any other time before that phone call.

Mum says she used to cry all the time when she was being courted by Dad, and unable to decide whether she, a Parsi, should marry him, a Muslim, a choice she had never anticipated having to make. Once she took her leap of faith, joy stepped into place. Maybe, for women, there is a time for tears, and then a time to put them away, because the men aren't crying and it appears unseemly.

Grief is a constant with me, more constant than depression, but tears are better controlled these days. When you rhyme the word 'tears' with 'scares', you understand tears are cuts, rents. Breaks. You were moving forward, then you started crying. Time stopped. Grief has a way of halting time. When we hear a person has died, our first question is, 'How old were they?' as though age has any bearing upon love. But humans have always lived through shifting patterns of mortality. We will not be halted for anything. Death, least of all.

I remember a phone call from my grandfather when I was ten. Dada was discoursing on the power of the mind and its relationship to white and red blood cells. He was on speaker, and his deep, modulated British-Simla accent filled the room. He was teaching me about healing. He was teaching me how to live.

I feel sure I was doing something else while my grandfather spoke. Maybe I was playing a board game with my brothers, but I must have been listening, carefully enough to have remembered and drawn on the teaching, several years later, when I needed it.

Dada had a weak heart fitted with a pacemaker. He was frail and gaunt when I knew him. An early accident had left him with shattered kneecaps, so he walked with a stick made from beautifully carved cherry-wood. He had silver hair and dreamy grey eyes softened by a faraway look. I could not imagine anyone gentler and yet I have learned from my mother that as a young man he was impatient, quick-tempered, vital. From father to grandfather, some men curve an unrecognisable arc. I can only be glad he was who he was, for me.

Dada died within months of our leaving India. My mother returned alone to Bombay to sit beside him in hospital and then, when he was wrapped in white and carried up the Zoroastrian Tower of Silence, she fell ill herself. In England, I was kicked out of drama class for sighing too loudly, too often. *If you are so bored, if we are boring you, then you can leave.* I retreated to the girls' bathroom. Someone found me there, later – maybe it was my drama teacher; I recall he was infinitely kind to me, afterwards. I was offered grief counselling but how can you talk to a stranger about someone you love? Someone you will never see again, in a country you will never call home again – not in the same way. Not in the old, easy way.

When I think about my grandfather, I think about his heart. And mine. I have tachycardia, which literally means 'swift heart'. There is little that can be done about my racing pulse, beyond a low dose of beta blockers, but it does make me listen more carefully to the syncopated rhythms of life and death resting between the beats of my heart. It also makes me think about heart attacks.

One night, on the ward, I am afraid to go to sleep. I am afraid to let my parents and brothers leave. What if I never wake up? I ask a registrar the next day, when I discover I am still alive, 'Can a heart give up because it's too tired? Are our heartbeats numbered?' He smiles, amused, and shakes his head. I'm not convinced. If our heartbeats are numbered, I'm worried mine are running out, run down, worn thin.

Do you ever think about your heart? Working away, unnoticed most of the time. Sometimes a shock of adrenaline sets up awareness, sometimes we pat our heart comfortingly, but unless you really listen to it, your heart remains a metaphor.

The day our dog Bruno died, he spent hours sky gazing out of the window on the second floor. Finally, he was cajoled downstairs, where he sat gazing at my mother, waiting for my father to come home from the hospital. It was late evening when Bruno finally laid his head upon Dad's feet and breathed his last.

Bruno has stayed with us in living and loved memory, so I knew from a young age that death did not mean oblivion. That if I died, I would go on existing in anecdote or the presence of a white butterfly, prancing on a summer's day. We know, instinctively, that we don't end at death. We know it through the practise of grief. We pull each other through. My grandfather has taught me more about death after his death than any book or spiritual teaching. He never left me. Even though I left him, left the country, wasn't there by his side when he died. It mattered to have his daughter by his side. And she was there.

I took my body away from India, away from our beloved house, Sandringham Villa, but most nights, my dreams return me there, to the rooms I still know best.

It isn't death we fear.

What we fear is the rapidity with which life closes over us. It happens so fast. One moment there are faces looking down on us, anxious, the next their attention is diverted by procedures that must be followed. Other people, doctors, lawyers, undertakers, intrude, well intentioned and purposeful. Your body must be disposed of. You are now a whisper no one can hear.

Here is the nub. We lose the body. That vehicle of miracles. The cluster of cells that move together in a dance. Instrument of music. Joke machine. Our children would miss us if we were gone. And so we fight to stay. And if with the fun and laughter comes the sorrow and conflict, we turn to art or commerce to distract us, to fulfil us, to make things to leave behind for a while.

Have you made a lot of money? an interviewer asks Bob Marley. 'How much is a lot?' he responds. 'I don't do it for the money. I do it for the people.' He was health conscious, watched what he ate and drank, exercised seriously. But when offered the chance to save his melanoma-stricken toe, he kept the toe and with that decision, allowed the cancer to slowly spread from toe to brain. But had he permitted the amputation of his toe, would it follow that he would still be alive today?

The sick person feels responsible for every single one of the losses incurred along the way. Guilty as a child who loses her new pencil case, ruins her only 'good' skirt. You were given the gift of life and all that it could entail and you betrayed that gift by losing the one thing that society heralds as its golden mantra: *health is wealth.* The rhythm of this particular guilt never quite leaves the chronically sick. It thrums beneath the surface of every social encounter and waits until you are alone to pounce. At worst a betrayal, at best a carelessness.

Some months ago, I dreamed my teeth were rotting and crumbling in my mouth. I looked it up on Google and experts claimed that such a dream, when analysed, is indicative of a loss of control, a feeling of helplessness. Things are falling apart. All true, all true, I mused sadly, and left it at that.

What I did not look at too closely was the possibility that my teeth really might be crumbling and the reason a very practical link to reality. I have been on steroids for almost twenty years and should have been eating slabs of calcium to survive the relentless degradation to my bones, my teeth and who knows what else. But I dislike the taste. No, worse, I hate it. The thick viscous chalk of it. The assault of almost two decades of illness related memories. Calcium is the husband I cannot divorce because of legal, political and religious reasons. But I cannot love him.

Picture a round tablet the size of a two-pound coin. As thick. Picture it white, and light. Place it on your tongue and bite. It will break. Some of it will crumble and a scent will emanate. Sweet, but sickly so. Your saliva will valiantly attempt successful mastication. It will ultimately fail, and you will need something to drink to wash the powder down. Do this twice a day for almost twenty years. In between, there will be other tablets that make you throw up, gag, bleed and burn with fever. In between, there will be heartbreak, loss and depression. All these will feed into the powdery scent, and one day you will not need to be in the same room as the chalk monster.

You will simply know where it is so you can avoid it.

No one will bother you in your avoidance. Calcium has become the very least of the doctors' problems. The doctors trust you to be maintaining yourself in these banal ways. You try the following ways:

Rates of Chew Speed: screw eyes tightly shut, hold breath and avoid slamming teeth on tongue in attempt to break imaginary world records of calcium chewing speeds. Speed cannot disguise taste. Time is treacle, and you will live inside the moment all day.

Crushed: you think it will somehow shrink in volume crushed, and thus be easy to disguise in a meal. Hot meals, cold meals, you even try soup. Lumps form, like unsieved flour. Your nose is not fooled.

Broken in half: and chewed hurriedly with a bite of chocolate fudge cake. Cake, on its own, begins to taste of chalk.

Broken into four quarters: your most gag-proof tactic. Each quarter systematically swallowed with a cup of tea, hot water, coconut water, juice. You do not know if efficacy is lessened by not chewing. You do not care. You still gag, and almost throw up but the thought of facing another eight pieces forces the triangle back down to do invisible work that you have disrespected for far too long.

When I write it out, when I am forced to think of my endless, daily dance of avoidance, I see it for the utterly meaningless act it is. I don't know how to take care of myself. It is a juggling act at all times. Concentrate your attention on one body part and three others fall apart. Escape the despair after this surgery or treatment and a new department enters, stage left. I am dancing on hot coals, feeling ridic-ulous but looking utterly stationary because everything is occurring so microscopically. I look like I ought to be juggling the acts everyone else is juggling – modern society has made jugglers of most of us – but I can't reach the usual objects to juggle. My arms are too full. Also, my legs lungs heart kidneys eyes bones blood. So, no husband baby job car.

Just as I am sensitised to depression, so I have been training myself to become sensitive to that which disconnects me from despair. Both are temporary in a way. But the second is a more useful skill to learn since the first is almost impossible to unlearn. Once you've tasted the worst of depression, you are always in danger of finding yourself there again.

Just as the triggers for depression are correct and present every day, so are the triggers for joy.

The scents that emanate from my mother's kitchen when she's making soup. Soup being cooked specifically for me because I am sick. Is chicken soup for the soul Jewish? Or universal?

The sound of my father's footsteps approaching my door. As the handle turns, a little smile turns up the corners of my mouth. It's almost a smirk. He loves me, I think, with a happy sigh.

The children are my best medicine. Or, at least, my most palatable one. Their energy seems inexhaustible and I get swept up in it. When I start to flag, we are usually near a bed somewhere in the house and I can devise a giggling game or a tickling game while I attempt a sneaky lie down (collapse in a heap). But they're on to me quick. *Get up, Shaista! Don't sleep. There's no time to waste.* It's not nothing, this being loved. It thrills me, ceaselessly.

I am not always cheerful. Why would I be? Whichever way you relate to hospital as an idea, is how it affects me in reality. I just have to find ways to navigate it; smiling or being cheerful and trying to relate on a human level is a coping mechanism. But it doesn't mean I have unlocked any sort of key to the matrix. I am too small a cog in the machinery of the NHS and, in the wider sense, within the social framework of being a person with chronic illness.

Most hospitals are usually a grey wash of a place. I've heard tell of children's wards being colourful places because we cannot bear our children to be both sick and unhappy. We are always amazed by the resilience of children and their capacity to be cheerful and smiling and brave in hospital, compared to their more miserable adult counterparts. Imagine if the adult sections of all hospitals were filled with cheery pictures, illustrations, bright pops of colour – well, perhaps not the fluorescent variety that currently graces Burger King's eating areas – but an equal measure of artistic and psychological research done into what makes humans happy and apply those images to hospitals.

Thinking positively is so much easier when you have help. Why else do we turn to our external devices to escape? We turn to our gadgets and gizmos, our bright little screens, to magic us away, anywhere from here. But it would be far better for our health, mental and physical, to be able to deal with the now, together, in hospital, without drawing on tremendous reserves of energy later, in isolation. Why are we left to our internal devices to switch on positivity and cheer?

Childhood, according to hospitals, ends at sixteen. I was eighteen when I was diagnosed. A rheumatologist wrote in my notes that, at nineteen, I needed to be more adult, take charge of my medical condition better, stop relying on my parents as much as I did. What on earth would he think of me now, twenty years later, living with my parents again, and still baffled by this octopus of a disease?

I feel a tenderness towards those who express their pity for me in this way: 'Oh Shaista, I feel for you. I wish things were different. I am so sorry you have to suffer in this way.'

There is something self-sacrificing about such words. They are offered to me without the usual requirement for balance expressed in this way: 'Come on! Cheer up! Try to be positive. Everyone has problems.' And then the exposition of that person's problems, or of something they read or saw in a documentary that makes my life with lupus appear a Disney film in comparison.

The second approach is perfectly human and justifiable.

But it is the first approach that moves me. It creates a bridge. It makes me want to reach out in any way I can to thank the person for their kindness in feeling pity for me; pity as their wish for mercy on my behalf. We associate mercy with its opposite: cruelty. We think of it in terms of justice and injustice.

But mercy as the milk of human kindness? As the genuine offering of solace, unasked, wanting nothing in return? Sweetness itself.

My mother offers me this kindness, this sweetness, more often than I deserve it. It is because of her ability to offer me this solace that I am able to offer her the solace of my smile, teary but unclouded. I feel better almost instantly when my mother says, 'Oh sweetheart, my darling, I wish you didn't have to suffer. I wish I could take your suffering away.' And because I know she means she would take it upon herself, and because I could not bear that, I cheer up. This suffering? What suffering? And I take the hand she is offering and together we cross over to the other side where it is greener for a while.

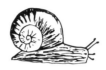

THE SOUND OF A WILD
SNAIL EATING

ome years ago, I happened upon a book called *The Sound of a Wild Snail Eating* by Elisabeth Tova Bailey.

I found myself reading Bailey's memoir on a plane and struggling to move past the first chapter. I wanted to stop time, rewind, and arrange to have a snail brought to me in the first months, first torments of my life with lupus. Bailey writes:

> *Illness isolates; the isolated become invisible; the invisible become forgotten. But the snail... the snail kept my spirit from evaporating. Between the two of us, we were a society all our own, and that kept isolation at bay.*

People often speak of the benefit of having a pet near you when you are ill, but a snail is not a pet. The snail probably had no conceptual image of Bailey as a human being, a woman, a patient recovering from a mysterious virus. But Bailey refers to the snail as 'my snail' within two days of its introduction into her life.

The Sound of a Wild Snail Eating is peppered with neat quotes from the likes of Rainer Maria Rilke, Kobayashi Issa, and this soothing couplet by John Donne:

And seeing the snaile, which every where doth rome,
Carrying his own house still, still is at home.

I read this book often, and slowly. Something about its very existence comforts me. I wish, from time to time, that I had written it. Other times I wish I were the snail. The snail knows itself. In its terrarium, it is master of a small kingdom. And, accordingly, behaves with the assured grace and dignity of a queenly king (snails being hermaphrodites). In the wild, the snail has predators, of course. But the snail seems unconcerned with these predators at random moments. Terror does not suddenly strike the snail during a gentle afternoon slither in slime. Does it?

Just as Bailey had slowness forced upon her, because a mysterious, bacterial pathogen resulted in severe neurological symptoms, so lupus has forced slowness upon me. Just as Bailey was bedridden, so have I been; the difference is in the length of the slowness visited upon us. A brief enforced Zen-monkish retreat can be endured by anyone and fruits of the nourished mind-body-soul can be harvested quickly. It is in the long laborious dragged out decades of a life with auto-immune disease that one's wisdoms and aphorisms are tested, repeatedly.

The paradox at the heart of my life is this: I want. I have an appetite for fame, money, success, happiness, friends, soul mates and children. But I am slow. I learn slowly. I put life teachings into practice, slowly. It takes me years to move from one spot to another. From one room to another. From one house to another.

I am lazy.

Even as I write that, I think this: I am not lazy. I am happy.

I had a decision to make about slowness when I was in the early years of living with lupus. Choose irritation, anger, frustration. Or choose contentment, happiness, awareness. With slowness, comes the full responsibility of making my life count every moment, because I am aware of every moment. I cannot escape into the running and the races which, until the coronavirus pandemic, constituted the lives of others.

There is a comfort in that race. The 'waking up, tumbling out, hating the morning but falling into it' routine. Your body moves before your mind commands it to. Bathroom, kitchen, children squabbling, marriage dynamic, carpool, email checks, ghastly work colleague, coffee, social media, social events, friends' needs, in-laws to dinner, weeding the garden, Pilates. Treadmill. Holidays.

I am permanently on holiday. Or in permanent retirement. I romanticise the working woman's life. I grieve for the mother I knew long ago I could never be: efficient, present every day and most important of all for a child's happiness and peace of mind – healthy. In other words, the mother I have been fortunate to have. I cannot speak for women who are mothers and are also battling disease and disability. They are heroic in ways I choose not to be, because it is a choice. Although I have now been officially diagnosed with multiple fibroids, I don't know for sure that I am gynecologically incapable of bearing children. What I do know is that I have been on cytotoxic drug therapies since I was eighteen. If I were to consider pregnancy, my life-saving therapies would be stopped immediately. I love children and love is the greatest requirement on the list of parent requirements. But not the only requirement. When I finally summoned the courage to discuss the possibility of pregnancy, my consultant was as honest with me as I had been vulnerable with her. This, she said, is what it would come down to: save my life or bring new life into the world at the risk of my own. Adopt alone and struggle alone. As the adoptive mother of three boys, she was speaking from an extremely informed and compassionate perspective.

One of the physical consequences of fibroids, is a belly that resembles cycles of pregnancy. I am in constant dialogue with this curious phenomenon of a body pushing outwards, appearing to nourish a phantom child, but containing only benign tumours within. I hold the shape, instinctively, in the way of all protective mothers-to-be. Learning to inject immunoglobulin serum into an already tender, distended abdomen was an additional trauma through the pandemic, until Dr. Kumar, my immunology consultant, gently suggested I switch the needling site to my thighs. Free of any reproductive associations, my thighs have served me well.

The last surgeon I spoke to, in his wisdom, did not recommend a hysterectomy, or even a myomectomy, as there was a possibility I might bleed out onto his table. *Lupus*, he said. *Blood clots, you know*. It was, of course, my decision, but… I thanked him, even as we both silently acknowledged the knowable barbarisms and the unknowable psychological landscape of womb cutting. And yet, even though my own body begs the question of me, to have children or not, to cut out my womb or not, I cannot bear to be told that I could have children if I really wanted because *there are ways*. I know there are ways, but it is not compulsory to bear children just because you are a woman. And because it is not compulsory, because I am under no legal or political obligation to bear children, I choose my life. I choose that freedom. I hate few things outside of outright cruelty and violence, but I do hate the way women without children of their own are backed into corners like cowering animals having to defend what is perceived to be a luxuriously empty nest. *Why is your nest empty?* asks society. *You could easily make room for more*. The woman without a husband or children is framed as a social magpie, picking at the family life of others, when if she had any sense of decency and virtue, she would concentrate on filling her nest with her own. This is a more acceptable and amusing framework for social conversation than acknowledging the real dangers and difficulties faced globally by girls and women from the moment of conception to labour and delivery. There are awareness movements and charities set up to educate, but the idea that women simply fall pregnant and reproduce is not only prevalent but, because of modern medicine, considered normal. Into the equation of a chaotic destructive immune system, the hopeless fragility of my eyes must also be accounted for. Only I know the full extent of the terrors of shadows and shrinking light.

What matters is that I have children in my life and that I have been considered worthy of being named godmother three times. I care deeply for the good opinion of my two sisters-in-law because they represent my ideal of womanhood. But I am also my ideal woman, because I live in conscious awareness of my freedoms. Freedoms that are not always visible or clear to others.

On my way to and from the BBC Cambridgeshire radio station, for an interview on World Book Day, I spend forty-five minutes with a driver named Dave. He had picked me up before: nothing uncommon about that, since, with my visual instability, I don't drive and have been using the same two taxi cab companies for twenty years. Some of these drivers have watched me grow up 'into a woman'. And this 'growing up into a woman' was the subject of Dave's discourse for approximately forty of the forty-five minutes to and from the radio station. Being the father of four daughters, he felt qualified to speak unequivocally and with authority on Young Women and Women in General.

Dave, at seventy, feels strongly that women lack confidence. A sentiment I agree with. Except I know that this lack of confidence is contextualised and justified in a sexist world. Dave seemed to have no source or context for his observations on the lack of confidence in the female sex. Yet, he joked, humourlessly, his wife had taken one look at him when he was a young, good-looking, up and coming political hot-head (his description of himself), and decided she was going to marry him. And that was that.

'Didn't you have any say in it?' I asked. (I felt I had to say something. He had just paused.)

'What do you think?' he faux grimaced.

'Yes,' I said. 'You did.'

He was undeterred. He complimented me several times over the course of the journey – on my face, my overall appearance, my manners, my diction. He proclaimed me nice, pleasant and clever, with the looks to (and this was what it was all leading to) Find A Man. 'If I was five years older than you,' he offered, as his ultimate accolade, 'your illness wouldn't put me off.'

I felt cornered as I always do in the confines of a small vehicle with a male driver who is taking a vivid interest in the creature he holds hostage. Dave, having set me up as a polite, clever, pretty woman who lacked confidence and needed to be told she was worth something, including his own male gaze and interest, forced me into a role-playing semblance of his creation. I became, with each word he uttered, the thing he saw. I found myself thanking him for his compliments. Politely. And when my mother called, I didn't pick up the phone, because that would have been impolite. She called again. I still didn't answer. Finally, when she called a third time, I woke up from the hypnosis of submission, wishing I could pull her physically out of the phone and into the seat beside me. 'I'm coming home to see you,' I said to her. Being able to say those words brought such comfort.

There are silences we participate in. Roles we submit to, rather than subvert. It takes energy, focus and discipline as much as it takes courage to speak out of turn because we don't see the traps we are in until it's too late. They snap shut on us, and then, in maddening circles of repetition, we find our voice. It takes years to build enough volume to break the trap. By which time, new traps have formed. There are recognisable patterns from my childhood memories of authority, uncomfortable rebellion and submission, that trace the tattoo of politeness by which I am guided. No matter what I think, or feel, this tracing is carved into me the way Braille dots have been hammered into my father's fingertips.

He can no sooner forget how to translate language into six raised spots than I can cease to be essentially polite. So, I imagine these conversations in taxis will continue indefinitely. Or, at least, until self-driving cars become a common reality.

When Immunology first asked me if I wanted to self-inject, I had just moved out of my parents' home and in to rented accommodation in a semi-private annexe called the Coach House. The thought of invading my first precious space of living as Independent Woman with weekly self-injections did not appeal. I wanted my rented space to be as free from needles and blood and bruising as possible. There was nothing I could do about the tablets and eye drops that spilled over surfaces to the floor, but on my tidy days, these could be neatly tucked into cupboards and drawers. Less easy to disguise syringes and the scent of anaesthesia.

It came as no surprise, once I had moved out of our home, that my mother regularly questioned whether I was eating at all. *I don't believe you*, she'd say, sounding a lot like Raf when he was two. I don't blame you, I'd think, stirring something vaguely food-like around a pan. My mother did not believe me capable of managing life on my own. A justified stance.

During my first year at university, shopping in Iceland for the usual meal-for-one ingredients, a woman accosted me at the exit doors. She had noticed me earlier and had no intention of letting me leave before she had her say. She whisked her hands around my face and body, and then pronounced that I had 'a yellow aura, a sickly aura' and that if I came with her to her house, which was only up the road, she would attend to my aura. I did not go unthinkingly. And that is all I can say in my defence. I went thinkingly. Knowingly. And yet, unstoppably.

The woman seemed elderly and harmless, if you can call a random supermarket aura-reader harmless. The other factor in her favour was the specificity of her identity. She was Parsi. Not just Indian, not just an Indian living in England, shopping in the same supermarket as me (there could have been several of those), but Parsi: one of the rare members of my mother's tribe. She had met me once before while I was with my mother, suspecting we were Parsis, and wanting to claim kinship. My mother had declined to be drawn into complicity by such manufactured claims, but respect for older members of the human race is drilled into the Indian child. Every older person is assigned honorary titles of 'Aunty' and 'Uncle' ensuring a kind of interconnected web of obligation or association.

Carrying my bags as well as hers up the lane, I was aware of a hummingbird singing a chorus of, 'Stupid girl! Stupid girl! Turn around *now*, stupid girl!' but my feet were walking in the opposite direction to my intelligence. I cannot recall the life history of this woman clearly. Suffice to say there were sensible reasons for her manifestation there. Her daughter was a graduate student at one of the Cambridge colleges. She was keeping house for her daughter. I remember the house. It was as though her flat in India had been transplanted, transmogrified here on an English street. I stepped back into a time before I knew time. I cannot remember much more. Perhaps she did attend to my aura. I seem to recall the figure of another woman in the shadows, but it is an unclear memory. I scuttled away as soon as was decently possible and never saw or contacted the duo again. I have survived many such encounters throughout my life. My yellow, sickly aura clearly does not put people off enough. Rather it draws them to me, thirsting for a thing inside me that I cannot see.

In the kitchen of my own, I turn the hob on, in preparation, and watch, horrified, as a plastic bag filled with rice that was casually resting on the surface, begins to burn and the cardboard egg container that had been resting beside it, begins to glow with the pretty sparkle of fire. I am, unfortunately, on the phone with my mother as this circus begins. I reach across the hob to switch the main power off, and my hand knocks the edge of the butter over. Two huge globes of butter fall onto the burning plastic rice paper concoction and melted rivers stream over the side of the oven into invisibility.

Do you want me to come over? my mother offers. *Shall I come now and help you clean up?*

No, I say. No, no, no.

I grab the handlebar of the oven, take a breath and pull. The whole structure comes away from the wall. Behind it is a disgusting mess of dirt and gritty gremlins left by the previous renter. But I can do this. I can clean up my own mess. My mother's voice, still anxious. My own voice, strangely calm. I've got this. This kitchen, though rented, is mine.

~

Was mine. I managed four years in the Coach House. I had moments of joyful freedom, writing in an upstairs window nook, and of being doubled over with the pain of loneliness, longing for more than the voices of my parents and nieces on the telephone. I was a ten-minute walk from them, and my feet began treading that path more and more often until one Christmas when, curled up in my mother's bed, I wrote my landlady a not altogether unexpected email. I was moving back home.

I take heart from the knowledge that Flannery O'Connor moved home to live with her mother and their many peacocks when lupus made her life untenable. And from the story of Maudie.

Directed by Irish director Aisling Walsh, *Maudie* depicts the unamorous coupling of Maud Lewis, the Nova Scotian painter, and her fish smuggling, peasant husband, Everett Lewis. Born with juvenile arthritis that eventually crippled her, she was betrayed by dishonourable family members who sold her precious newborn for money, telling Maud that her baby had been born deformed like her mother, and buried

LUPUS, YOU ODD UNNATURAL THING

immediately.

Years later, Maud learns the truth. Everett takes her to see her baby, now a grown woman, happy, tending to roses outside the white and blue shutters of her home. Maud cowers in the shadows of her husband's truck, broken and healed, simultaneously.

The shadows of Maud's life were painted over by her extraordinary capacity for wielding joy into simple brushwork. Deceptively simple, her work began to sell, began to be loved, was commissioned by the likes of Richard Nixon, then President of the United States.

By the end of her life, Maud was crippled with arthritis, unable to walk, but still able to hook her brush into the curled claw of her hand and do the thing that made her utterly content with her life. Paint pictures. The whole world framed in a tiny square of happiness.

In my own little cabin in the garden – 'The Shanny', so named for the young mother (Sharon) and her baby boy (Danny) for whom this little house was originally built – I have been wielding my brushes and paint. Every dark or gloomy corner now has a fresh white, blue or pink coat, reassuring my eyes of light.

To be an artist is to know suffering, but to know beauty and joy, more.

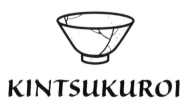

KINTSUKUROI

When the demolition of the Ayodhya mosque sparked national religious riots in December 1992, my brothers and I were told to say our goodbyes to school and friends, and within a week, we had boarded a plane for England.

Within months, India had calmed herself, and Bombay was safe again, but our lives had already changed, irrevocably. Intending to keep our connection to India vital, our parents sent the three of us back to Bombay during every English school vacation.

It took three trips for the disease to take hold of me. Each time I went, I suffered a little deeper the strange new role of outsider. Our precious home, Sandringham Villa, had been sold to a family so rich they had gilded parts of the house. Gone was the crumbling, old world beauty of the garden and balconies. The friends I usually stayed with had been our neighbours, so the temptation to visit the old treads was always too strong to resist. Trauma layered into trauma each year as I walked up to a house, which was no longer my home, crying so hysterically that the chowkidars looked embarrassed. I could feel their pity. *Who is this girl, and why can she not stop crying?*

I remember spending my last days of that third trip, throwing up, and my friend's mother comforting me. I remember a fever beginning to grow and wanting only my mother. I remember the sweet relief of

having an aunt who worked for Air India, conjuring her magic so fast
that I was on a plane before I knew it, travelling alone, burning up, but
going home, away from home, home.

Ever since that summer of 1997, I have been hesitant to return to India
because I didn't want to return ill.

But I have returned, twice.

In December 2014, I visited Rizwan, who was living and working
in Bangalore. For seventeen years, I had dreamed of my return to India;
I had assumed it would be Bombay I returned to. I thought Bombay
would be the Real Return, so I tried, twice, to return 'home' from
Bangalore. The first time, my flight was cancelled on the morning of
my departure, and on the next occasion, I awoke to a fever. As I lay
in a heap of sweaty tachycardia, I realised I was already home. In my
brother's home, I am home. The twins were not disappointed by my
change of plans.

On the last night of the year, the rains came and washed away the
remains of our old selves. In the morning, I went downstairs and sat in
the garden for a few moments. A cluster of sari and bangle clad women
gardeners wove a circle around me. They were off in the distance one
moment, and the next were crouching inches from my feet. One lady
asked me the time – maybe she really needed to know. Or maybe she
just wanted to hear me speak, make a connection. We didn't speak the
same language – I was in the south of India, where the food, languages
and pace of life are different from the north. But the smiles are the same.

I ended the old year and began the new year re-reading Thich
Nhât Hanh's *Fragrant Palm Leaves*, the memoir he wrote at thirty-six,
the same age I was. He wrote the book in New Jersey and Princeton,
while in exile from Vietnam, not knowing his exile would continue
until his seventieth year. Or that he would have a stroke in his eightieth

year, which would leave him comatose. A few days into 2015, I heard the news that Thây was no longer in a coma. He had opened his eyes, was responding with chuckles to humorous stories, was breathing, was re-learning how to drink a cup of tea.

Most mornings in Bangalore, I would hear birds, and someone would begin the onerous task of sweeping dust. Dust in India cannot be swept away. It can be swept from here to there, but mostly it fluffs itself up in the air and lands daintily again by the sweeper's feet, as though to suggest they would both be more comfortable if they could just accept what they are to each other. Dust provides the sweeper with a job. And the sweeper provides dust with excitement, a little flurry, a change of pace and place.

Why is dust? It is not pretty or useful.

Why is illness? It is not pretty or useful. And yet here I am, dusty with illness, and that ubiquitous, meaningless word, pain.

And yet here I am, loved.

I am *kintsukuroi*, broken pottery joined by gold dust and lacquer. While I was in Bangalore, a friend of mine sent me an image of such a bowl made more beautiful by its interesting narrative; the kintsugi philosophy made me think of my broken pieces joined not by stitches and scar tissue, but by the gold dust of love and friendship.

As the days passed, and my return to winter in England drew nearer, I began to understand that I carry home with me wherever I go. I am home wherever I am. When my parents packed Sandringham Villa into crates and the trucks arrived outside our new English home, furniture that had travelled seas to be with us brought the old stories with them. Persian carpets, teak carvings, sandalwood statues, took up residence beside daisies, geraniums and poinsettias. In the early years, when English school friends visited, I felt embarrassed by our furniture, which seemed an obvious manifestation of how different we were – their homes looked nothing like ours. But I am a writer, a lover of stories, and such embarrassments faded quickly, replaced by my original love for Sandringham, the house that continues to breathe life into my dreams.

I returned once more to my brother's home in Bangalore, four years later, for my fortieth birthday. And this time I did venture north. For three days. Twenty-one years after leaving the city of my birth, I had courage (and calendar space between Bangalore and Singapore, or more accurately, between Eva-Ellie and Bella-Raf) for only three days. I met as many of my dear friends as I could and walked as much of the loved land as I could with the hours beating time. And cried with exhaustion at each day's end. If I return once more, I hope to unfurl with the slowness of my life in England. I hope to do nothing, on a balcony, listening to crows and drinking coffee. I want to be driven inside by the rain. I want to remember what it felt like to read a book in the noisiest, most populous city in the world, and hear only my imagination. Three days were long enough, though, to remind me I live outside of time wherever I am. A different clock runs through me always, counting breaths of pain, and breaths of sorrow, even as I chirp and muster my semblances of normal.

It has been the strangest year. A pandemic shook the globe free of its frame, and a new language began to be learned. My cousin asks if I have been writing lots of poetry. It strikes her that there is poetry in this, this time of strangeness, of discovering one's ability to adapt – the beauty inherent in that. And indeed, Carol Ann Duffy initiated a project titled 'Write Where We Are Now', gathering the thoughts and feelings of her fellow poets on our global viral tidal wave. We surprise ourselves with adaptation, and it thrills us to discover – still here, still here. No matter what. Tsunami, earthquake, the plague, coronavirus. The Great Depression, the Wall Street Crash, demonetisation. The end of circuses, the beginning of Tiger King. The end of letter writing, the beginning of emoticons. Lose limbs, become an Olympic athlete. Hospital a dangerous place? Self-inject.

What gets lost in the adaptation? The transition. The nuances within those transitions. My anxiety before the sub cut training, my sleepless nights. My terrible sense of the cold once I had penetrated my flesh, in two different sites, slowly, each ml a painful new reality. You'll get used to it. Some people love it. You won't even feel it. Later, someday. You'll be like the others. Who smile and laugh and brush this off. It's nothing. Nothing. Nothing.

The extremely vulnerable must continue to isolate. It is for their own protection. Meanwhile, we rush to open our vital economies. Our schools. Life must be returned to normal. Meanwhile, there is a rush on Hydroxychloroquine. India closes her borders to exporting the raw materials. Poor lupus patients. Meanwhile, it's possible that doesn't matter because being on immunosuppressive therapies may explain why auto-immune patients aren't dying, en masse. You're fine, lupus patients. Your cytokine storms aren't as wild and intemperate as ours. As you were. But all the same, stay home afterwards. After our storms subside. Our bodies are the frontlines. We will protect you. We may also infect you. Just stay quiet. With that needle in your flesh. It is for your own good. The front door is your safest bet. Behind that front door... well, never mind that.

That sense of cold I mentioned? It is the place of loneliness, of abandonment. Of being protected for one's own good under strictly controlled guidelines. Of the new normal being the old normal, only with an edge. But it must be contained, or else our little cup of sunshine will be consumed with the single thought that threatens to destroy us on any ordinary day. The lupus patient was never meant to survive.

And yet she does, with a paintbrush in her hands. Where poetry fails me, I paint my reality. Back and forth. Wax on, wax off. Until I become something akin to the Buddhist novice, who, in elevating a simple monotonous task with consciousness, finds nirvana.

I used to fantasise about the nunnery. It was always my safe place, my safe word, for a future when things fell apart. No money, no husband, no children, no independence? No problem. Prayer would hold me still. In some wooden crevice, peace. Repeated ad infinitum.

Then I met nuns. Going into seclusion, coming out of monastic life. Either way, they were going into battle. It is all a battle. Even peace. At the last resort, Thích Quảng Đức set his body alight. Martin Luther King Jr. was shot from a distance. Mohandas Karamchand Gandhi was shot, three times, point blank, face to face with his killer, Godse.

For years leading up to and then after the Molteno tube implant, I had an imaginary gun nestled at the corner of my left eye. I learned to live with it, wake and sleep in conscious awareness of it. I used all the tricks, visualising its transformation into petals, kisses, love, until one day it disappeared. Manifesting somewhere else, I presume, in someone else's psyche. I say I am kintsukuroi not because I know I am made beautiful, but because I hope such beauty can be possible. Are we not all broken and scarred in some places? Then are we not all made beautiful?

As my birthday once again draws near, the white butterflies are beginning to gather for the dance. I hear leaves crackle. There's someone out there. I look up and squint into the sun. Black strands of hair fall protectively across my eyes.

A memory comes to me, of words I wrote when I was twenty.

I am behind the curtain, breathing ever so slightly,
watching the wind rip the grass
and sunlight dance through my hair,
making chestnut waves in a black rainbow.

I knew myself then. I know myself now. And what of the self to come? I can't see her when I look directly for her. But I can feel her watching me. I can hear her, listening, waiting. She knows I will not let her fall. Palms out-stretched, we hold on to each other.

Just hold on.

WE ARE A WEBSITE

In the packed waiting room of the blood test department, I found myself sitting beside a man in his seventies or eighties. I was in my twenties at the time.

As our conversation unfolded, he wanted to know if I was married, what I was studying or doing for a living. I had been in the throes of a long, slow flare, my glaucoma operations were around the corner and I was in between degrees. I told the stranger the truth: I was a girl with a serious illness, which prevented me from living a 'normal life'. The man's response was quick, angry and bordering on repulsion. 'Never,' he remonstrated, 'never tell anyone what you have just told me. You are a beautiful girl, you look completely normal. If you hadn't told me, I would never have known.' This point seemed particularly to bother him. I had destroyed his illusion of me. The fact that we were both in a hospital, waiting for our blood to be drawn, seemed to have escaped his notice.

Afterwards, sorting through and past the shame he had deliberately inflicted on me, I settled on anger. I am an ornery character; born in that moment was a firm conviction to ignore his instruction and, in fact, do precisely the opposite. I didn't know at that time that one day I would create a blog with the word 'Lupus' written boldly across the header. Or that I would write a book detailing my life with a serious, invisible illness that some people would rather pretend doesn't exist.

If I were diagnosed today, I would be entering a ready-made world of communication and connection. I would probably already have a Facebook, Twitter or Instagram account. I might have created a Tumblr or a blog, just to trial my voice in the magnificent unknown that seems able to support all our writings. When I was diagnosed in August 1997, I turned to the place I had always lived, the blank page, and continued my conversation with myself. With each year that rolled me along, a new journal would appear and once completed, step onto the shelf along with its predecessors. When I began my blog in 2009, it seemed the most un-Shaista thing I could do, but the thing that felt like it belonged to Other People, out there in the world of technology, soon became the clearest expression of myself and my deepest connection to others. There were no Others. There was only us. For richer, for poorer. In sickness and in health. We make the official vows out loud to one other person, but we embody those vows for everyone. We are devoted to being here, on earth, united by our desire to not die.

So much of what I write is in direct response to what I am reading. My becoming and being a writer is in direct response to my being a reader, but much of what I write is also in direct response to what I am watching. Some people use music as a soundtrack to their writing. I use film. When I lay in my bathtub a decade ago contemplating the nature of self-annihilation, I did that other thing human beings do when they are looking into the face of their extinction. I searched for what would make me want to stay. In times of the fiercest depression, our loved ones are not a reason to stay. To release them from our masked, haunted eyes, we would do anything. The answer that came to me might seem callous and superficial to you. But here it is: movies.

Movies have always been a source of joy and education. I think I've seen every film that might come under the heading of 'Inspiring' from *Dead Poets Society* to *Schindler's List* to *Amélie* and *Lion*. I will admit I haven't seen *Rocky* yet. Film has always been a source of travel for me, as it is for billions of us, certainly for the large portion of a billion Indians, who transcend their daily struggles with cinematic escapism. For me, Mira Nair's *cinéma vérité* appeals more than the glitz of Bolly, Holly and Nollywood because I am constantly trying to learn things as well. I am fascinated by the small revelations made by creators like Emma Thompson discussing the history behind her screenplay of *Sense and Sensibility*. How long it took. How many drafts. If it weren't for the extraordinary platform that YouTube provides, I would be ignorant of such revelations.

A few years into the writing of this book, an online journal published my essay on my experiences in the Patient Short Stay Unit. The name of the journal was 'We Are A Website'. When Clive read the title in an early draft of this memoir, he immediately approved. He liked the idea of the modern human race being a website, each of us plugged into the matrix. It also appealed because one of the last activities he poured energy into, aside from his ongoing books of poetry and last volume of memoirs, was his own website.

The first time we met, Clive was unamused that I had not read his poetry. I didn't know he was a poet. I had barely recognised him. To correct this clear failing on my part, he directed me to his website. *Take a look at it, kid.* Clive was partial to the notion that I would be his Young Person Advocate, extolling his literary virtues to the new and hopelessly Clive-deprived generation. I failed in this, because I didn't like the idea that anything I wrote about the critic, would have the critic critique it first. Case in point: I blogged about our first encounter over Marian Keyes' cake. Clive read it and decided I needed to amend the bit where it suggested he had smiled at me first. 'You smiled first, or I would never have done. Change that bit.' I did change it. Not because of who smiled first, but because I was the one who dragged her pump across the ward and offered a slice of Guinness and malt cake.

'The ego arranges the bad light to its own satisfaction' Clive wrote in my poetry journal of that time, quoting himself from his first bestseller, *Unreliable Memoirs*. We discussed our favourite poets. I think I read one of my poems aloud to him. My poems were 'pretty things' to Clive, but he assured me I had a long way to go. Clive's patronage of me was always affectionate, and not easily rebuffed because of the simple truth of his fame compared to my continuing wildflower under a rock status. *Keep at it, kid. I do have a few years on you, you know.* The patronage took a turn after Clive invited me to a poetry launch party at Pembroke College, his alma mater. I got into a small debate with one of Clive's friends about the fact that *Cultural Amnesia*, which records a hundred lives in detail, focuses on only ten women. Not very feminist in my book. 'Clive's the least sexist man you'll ever meet,' said his friend, staunchly. Hard to argue with a pal of Clive's in a room filled with pals of Clive's. Nonetheless, the next time we were hooked up to the drips, Clive mentioned he'd been writing to his friends about how thoroughly he was enjoying educating the young woman they had met at the party. 'I educate myself,' I said, a hint of the Arctic about me. He never spoke of educating me again. Rather, it was I who seemed to be educating him, once, when I mentioned Queen Bey (we were discussing Taylor Swift and Tom Hiddleston at the time). He promised to go look up Queen Bey when he got home. 'Twerp!' he rushed off in an email that evening. 'You ought to have told me Queen Bey was Beyoncé!'

We didn't agree on certain global matters and we were placed very differently on the scale of the white patriarchy, which lent much of our interaction during the MeToo year a fraught tension, palpable only to me, I suspect. What we did agree on, was the danger we were both in. Clive's eyes always lit up when he saw me walk on to the ward, and my gladness at seeing him, and exchanging a little repartee, was too marked to mean anything other than here was a friend, whose tomorrows were not guaranteed. The carcinomas were chomping away at Clive's face, skull, ears. Although he was complimentary about my book, he felt my ending was lacking something. He voiced this to my mother one day when she came to fetch me from the ward. *You have a talented daughter. It's a good book she's got there. We just need to do something about that ending, make sure people know how much danger she is in.* Later that evening, an email pinged in with apologies for his ineptitude. Telling my mother that her daughter needed to spell out for her reader that she was going to die, and perhaps soon, was ill-considered.

In all likelihood, his own death stood guard over every sentence he wrote. *Your readers will be only too happy to forget the danger you're in, kid.* He meant they'd forget me. He meant they'd forget him.

I think of it this way. If my reader has come to the end of my book, I am amazed and gratified. Thank you for staying with me, so close beside me. I have no desire to frighten you here, as we walk towards the end, together.

And yet, Clive's warning is all too knowing; he was, after all, the man who observed human foibles and turned all of us into reality TV aficionados capable of an almost dispassionate commentary on the lives of others. Without enough drama, stories like mine, lives like mine, are too easily subsumed in the 'But You Don't Look Sick Therefore Perhaps You Aren't Sick' conundrum.

To this day, I get handed business cards at the hospital by people wanting to help because I look an oddity; younger than my years, I look like I ought to be living a different life. One they will help me live, if only I give them a chance.

No, you don't understand, I want to tell them. This life? This dear, precious life? It is mine to interpret, unravel and tend to. Thank you for your offer, but here, take my book instead. I have written my life for you so you can see how beloved I am to myself. I know every thread. I have held each one – the delicate, the fire, the steel – and quilted them into something tangible. Proof of life. A beautiful life.

Many years after the Molteno, Keith asked me to participate in a conference at the John Van Geest Centre for Brain Repair at the University of Cambridge. 'Just a handful of people in jeans' was how he had sold the event to me, to dispel my anxiety. At the brain institute, Keith introduced me with images of my damaged optic nerve, my tortured disc and scar tissue, so the last thing the scientists were expecting was a perky fashion plate, who tripped up the stairs to the stage, picked up her mic and gave a sweeping wave, as though she'd spent years waving at an audience of hundreds. Keith had promised that the researchers would be more nervous than I would be, and to forgive them any insensitive blunders. He was possibly right about the first, I wouldn't presume so, but they didn't commit the second. In fact, I was asked the question that enabled me to reveal my true self: *did writing poetry help me survive the onslaught of the disease?* The questioner, I later discovered, turned out to be the director of the brain institute. At the time, I simply thought him an insightful human being.

Today, type anything of interest into YouTube and you will find a person living a close semblance of your life. Yes, an edited version, but still, lived. Vlogs are our new portals into each other's lives. You can keep up with what someone is enduring or enjoying a matter of hours after the event if the vlog is edited, or immediately, if it is being live streamed. And even though there is no scriptwriter or Hollywood glamour, or rather because there is no script or glamour, we are drawn in, to the authenticity of the act of love. Sharing is an act of love. Here, you see this? This is me. The moment you start questioning, 'Why should anyone care?' you lose the will to record another episode of your life.

You must simultaneously find the will to believe you are worth being seen, being cared for and, also, believe being unseen doesn't equate to being unloved.

Although, perhaps it does? If love is understanding, and under-standing requires visibility, then perhaps we do need to be seen to be loved. The first time my life with lupus became visible to others was when I made it deliberately visible with blog posts documenting my days in hospital while I was living them. I bestowed an authority and an authenticity upon myself with the voice that emerged as my blog grew. The first time I had a picture taken of me in hospital was a year and half later. It is of me smiling, posed with the book of poetry I was writing in that day, fully aware, fully conscious and happy because I had walked into the ward that morning and would be walking out, the same evening. It was a deliberate decision, asking the senior ward nurse to photograph me in the Patient Short Stay Unit, sitting in the giant blue faux leather armchair while the IV tube dripped a clear liquid into me. 'Why do you want to take a picture in here?' asked Annamma, unde-cided on whether to indulge me or bleep a doctor to check my sanity.

On another occasion, I decided to drive her even crazier by adopt-ing a martial pose, in the Go Ju Ryu style of Karate, open hands, knees bent, head slightly tilted, ready for the kick. 'Are you mad?' asked Annamma, her Keralan accent heightened by stress and annoyance. 'Gone crazy? I'm not taking this photo!' The ward was empty apart from the two of us, and at the desk, maybe one other nurse, shaking her head at my antics. 'Come on!' I admonished. 'Quick!' Before my sense of the ridiculous failed me, or my ability to be a karateka after eight hours of chemotherapy. Annamma took the picture, but it is blurred. Because she was laughing and scolding me, and I was laughing and scolding her.

To this day, I have only a handful of pictures of myself in hospital, because although times have changed and we make little distinction between that which must not be photographed and everything else that can, it never occurs to anyone in my family to photograph their sick daughter or sister while she is hooked up to tubes and recovering from the latest surgical intervention. When I asked my mother to photograph me after eye surgery, her response was not dissimilar to Annamma's. Later, on Facebook, my friends commented on how beautiful and peaceful I looked, black hair splayed out against crisp white pillows, a half-smile on my lips, despite the bandaged eye. How brave I looked! they said.

My mother sees none of this. She sees a hospital gown, unbrushed hair, and her daughter suffering. She feels the weight of the memory of minutes ticking by as she waits alone, unable to see what the surgeon is doing to her child's already scarred and damaged left eye. To appease her, when we return home, I tell her to take a picture of me near a flower bed in our garden, smiling, in a bright yellow top, hair brushed, bandage off. It doesn't appease her. I still have a clear eye patch on, and she still sees the suffering. But it is too late. I am too aware of the power of the visual for those who do not live a life like mine.

The photographs, occasional though they are, have made an aspect of my life in hospital accessible to friends and blog readers in a way that words cannot. See? See me? Here I am, this is me. This too can be endured with grace.

⌒

The last taboo for a woman telling the story of her life is to admit to self-love. To confess that she needs only the glory of her own company to make her happy. Alice Walker puts it perfectly:

Womanist: Loves music. Loves dance. Loves the moon. Loves the Spirit. Loves love and food and roundness. Loves struggle. Loves the Folk. Loves herself. Regardless.

I am the subject of *my* life, the subject of *my* book, *my* blog. At the heart of healing lies this question: *Do you love you?* Yes. Yes, I do.

The courage required of me isn't contained in the suffering glimpsed at through the images of my life; it is in the act of sharing.

Here I am, this is me. Do you care? I take a leap of faith to believe you do.

Coda

Fire and clay and brimstone;
something has changed in me.

Hands have wrought through
and through me.

I am changed;
I am becoming

something I once knew
would be me.

ACKNOWLEDGEMENTS

As I mention in 'The Appointment in Samarra', I began this book in 2013, so there have been many readers along the way. I have appreciated every offering of time and advice. Irfan and Rizwan, my brothers, were my first and final major contributors to the shape and tone of this book. Perveen and Chotu, our parents, to whom this book is dedicated, are the reason I keep the faith. To Colette, my sub cut companion and stalwart zebra, and to my doctors, Keith, Paul and Kumar, who lent their real names and spirits to my endeavour – I am grateful for you.

And finally, to my sisters, Theresa and Angelina, for loving me, and giving me four perfect beings to adore – my beloved Rafi, Bella, Eva and Ellie.

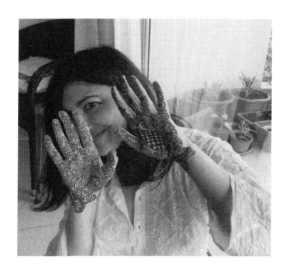

ABOUT THE AUTHOR

Shaista Tayabali was born in Bombay, India, and now lives and writes in Cambridge, England. She is the author of two poetry collections, *Something Beautiful Travels Far* and *Two Women,* and creator of the blog *Lupus in Flight* www.lupusinflight.com. She is currently working on her first novel.

Printed in Great Britain
by Amazon